Silent Grief, Healing, and Hope

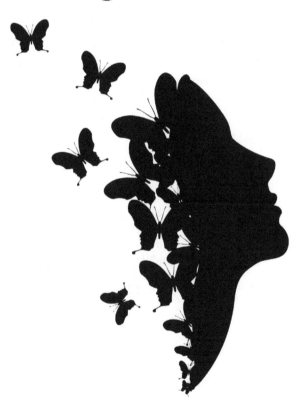

Compiled by Danielle Lynn

Disclaimer

This book is for inspirational purpose only. The views expressed in this book are based on the author's own personal experience or the outcomes with clients that they may have personally witnessed. Although we have made every reasonable attempt to ensure accuracy in the content of this book, we assume no responsibility for errors or omissions in the information provided. The compiler, publisher and authors do not assume any responsibility or liability whatsoever on the behalf of the purchaser or reader of these materials.

For more information, visit:

Publisher: Your Shift Matters Publishing, a Division of Dana Zarcone International, LLC www.danazarcone.com

Graphics and Editing by: Amanda Ni Odhrain www.letsgetbooked.com

Formatting by: Bojan Kratofil www.expertformatting.com

ISBN: 978-1-5136-5450-8

Gratitude

I want to express gratitude and appreciation to the other women in this book! I wanted to compile a pregnancy loss and infertility book because of my own struggles and lack of awareness and education on these topics. Without my co-authors, this book would not exist. Vulnerability was needed for these sensitive and meaningful stories. These women are brave, strong, loving individuals who opened their hearts to the world. I cannot thank these women enough for their participation in this book!

I want to thank my publisher for saying "YES" to this anthology! I had a vision and knew I had chosen the right person to teach me the ropes and guide me. It's an honor to call you my friend and I love you! Thank you for your guidance, leadership and ongoing support of my writing and publishing!

I want to thank our editor Amanda for her leadership. Your dedication and patience with all of us has made this journey possible. Our stories expressed a lot of grief and confusion, and your way with words helped to bring them to life! I appreciate your hard work and support.

I want to express love and gratitude to my husband, Darren. Our journey is in this book for the world to read and feel inspired. Your love, support, and openness mean so much to me. I love you with my whole heart and I know I am blessed to have you as my spouse, partner, best friend, and husband. My life has been better with you in it! We got this, no matter what!

Table of Contents

Foreword

I met Danielle at a conference that was geared towards helping women raise their influence in their respective businesses. There were so many women attending that conference but she and I clicked immediately. There was something about her calm presence and warm smile that made her stand out. We sat next to each other for the duration of the conference and while there wasn't a lot of time to get to know each other we stayed in contact and our friendship has continued to blossom.

Soon after the conference ended, I learned that Danielle had suffered multiple miscarriages. My heart hurt for her. How could someone who was so kind and giving experience so much pain? It didn't seem fair. She had every reason to give up and feel defeated after enduring so much devastation. Instead, she has chosen to channel her pain into a beautiful gift which is the book you are now reading.

Danielle sought out women who have experienced the struggle with infertility along with those who have endured a miscarriage or child loss. She chose to be brave and help others who were silently struggling. She wanted to create a place where women could share their stories in an effort to heal but also create a resource for women who were grieving behind closed doors.

This book was created in an effort to serve the women who have experienced fertility issues or miscarriage and are trying to heal emotionally or physically while harboring feelings of shame and guilt. For those women who are silently grieving after the loss of a child or because they are having difficulty becoming pregnant. For women who feel like they are alone and desperately need some comfort. And for women who are struggling with the reality that they may never give birth to a healthy baby.

Thank you, Danielle, for creating this compilation in an effort to help others. You have taken your pain and grief and turned it into something beautiful. You are a true inspiration and I am so lucky to call you my friend!

To the beautiful woman reading this, you are not alone on this journey. You are loved, you are strong, you are brave and I hope that you always remember there are women out there who love you and will support you!

Amy McNally
www.coachamymcnally.com
coachamymcnally@gmail.com
Facebook Group: The Joyful Entrepreneur

Introduction

This book has found its way into your hands for a good reason. Whether you are struggling with infertility, had a miscarriage, or experienced a pregnancy loss, I hope this book brings you comfort and hope. You are not alone!

My struggle to have a child of my own is the reason why this book exists. Growing up, I never really thought about having a child or being a mom. I have always been focused on my own personal goals, relationships, and career, but I began missing something in my life. When I began a serious relationship with my husband, I knew what it was. I wanted to have a child, not just a baby. I wanted to have a family. This hit me hard when I knew I found my other half. I feel this part of my life is not only about what it means to be a parent, but who I would co-parent with.

The journey to becoming a mother has not been easy. My husband and I have lost three babies through miscarriages and I had a miscarriage in my first marriage. Part of my grief is speaking with other women, other mothers, and compiling this book. I am learning more about the grieving process as I walk with these women on this journey of infertility and pregnancy loss. There is no way around grief, and it does not matter when it begins.

I have struggled for years to find a resource that would speak to me about infertility and pregnancy loss. A place to share relatable stories, education, and awareness about our struggles and heartache, while providing hope and support. Last year I began researching pregnancy loss books, writing inspirational stories, and having my work published. When looking for pregnancy loss books, I found very limited resources and support in my local bookstores and online. This led me to wanting to provide personal stories, with a community of women that unfortunately shared the same heartache; infertility, miscarriage or pregnancy loss stories.

I believe this book will *inspire* you with reading the heartfelt stories of these women, in being able to relate to their experiences and journey of motherhood! I *know* this book will provide medical knowledge and give you guidance in what to request to your doctors with bloodwork, fertility testing, and sonogram images! I feel this book will provide you *comfort* through the grief and loss of losing a child or trying to conceive!

I wish I had this book during my miscarriages and struggles to become pregnant, instead of the internet and Dr. Google. These stories are real! These women are real! These struggles are real! The lessons learned are from the authors' heart and experiences. The statistics are high and continue to climb!

I know this book will bring awareness to the struggles with conceiving, experiencing infertility issues, and pregnancy loss.

Much love,
Danielle Lynn

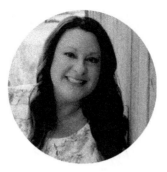

Danielle Lynn

Danielle Lynn, originally from New Castle Pennsylvania, resides in East Palestine, Ohio with her husband. Danielle earned a Bachelor of Science degree through Slippery Rock University and holds a Master's Degree in Social Work through the University of Pittsburgh. She is currently a Christian coach and an addictions counselor in Pennsylvania as well as a bestselling author on Amazon.

Danielle had her first solo publishing experience in 2019 with an inspiration planner, focusing on the teachings of gratitude and personal photography. With these publishing's Danielle has reconnected with her alumni, Slippery Rock University, having her publishing's featured in the university bookstore. Danielle's published works can also be found at Leana's Bookstore in Hermitage, Pennsylvania.

Even with a busy career, Danielle has many hobbies and interest. Danielle enjoys being outdoors, spending time with her family and friends, relaxing with her pets, antiquing, woodworking, reading, writing, cooking, and taking motorcycle rides with her husband.

Connect with Danielle:
www.daniellelynninspires.com
www.Instagram.com/dschotzie

Danielle Lynn Inspires Community:
https://www.facebook.com/groups/805852296449085

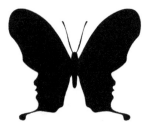

Front Row Seat with Jesus

By Danielle Lynn

So here I am today, wondering if I'll ever become a mother.

I feel complete panic and anxiety over the topic of becoming pregnant again. I have been through my share of testing and doctor's appointments. I have had countless blood tests (one sitting required seventeen vials!), fertility testing to check the lining of my fallopian tubes and uterus, numerous D&C's and still…. I have no answers.

Pushing myself to find the right doctors has been very difficult. Worrying about the next emergency room visit makes me want to avoid those doctor visits. Dealing with physical pain, emotional pain, grief, and loss has been difficult. I expect a doctor to tell me I should stop trying to conceive because it would be unhealthy to keep trying to have a baby. This hasn't happened. Not one doctor has told me it would be in my best interest to stop trying to have a child or recommend treatment past Clomid. Clomid was recommended by a fertility doctor a couple of years ago to help produce healthy eggs for reproduction because I am over the age of thirty-five. Did you know that at the age of thirty-five doctors describe women as being in an "advanced maternal age?"

I have a fear of attachment during each pregnancy because of the end results. While I am currently not pregnant and still working through my emotions, I have learned so much about myself, and

I want others to know that you are not alone. The statistics for infertility issues and reoccurring miscarriages are extremely high; we need to break the stigma and keep talking.

All my miscarriage experiences have been completely different, but the outcome has been the same. I am left heartbroken, unable to hold my child, celebrate birthdays or any holidays, watch them have their first day of school, watch my husband teach him or her new things, and watch them grow to be adults. When you're pregnant, all these visions and dreams come into your thoughts.

In my first pregnancy, I miscarried twins almost exactly a month apart, in my first trimester. This was in my first marriage. When I first became pregnant, I remember feeling extremely nervous. I was in my mid-twenties, not really prepared to be a mom mentally and emotionally, although I was extremely excited! I envisioned how I was going to tell my parents that they were going to be grandparents. I feel this is a normal reaction, especially when you have a close family. I felt this way with every pregnancy but of course, after each loss, you become less excited and more nervous about making the announcement.

Three of my last miscarriages have happened more recently, and I am now forty-three years old.

My husband and I got married on May 20th, 2017. The same week we had gotten married, I found out I was pregnant, but after our wedding nuptials. All week I was feeling nauseous and lightheaded. I thought these symptoms were due to my nervousness and excitement in getting married! A few days after the wedding, after the busyness of the ceremony and visits with family and friends had calmed down, I began to just "feel" pregnant. It is hard to explain why I honestly thought I might be pregnant but it just hit me one day! So I bought a home pregnancy test. Well, not one test, a few home pregnancy test! I was in complete shock when I saw how fast all the test became positive! Instantly I became nervous! Nervous about telling my 'new' husband and thinking, *Is this seriously happening, right now?* I was also thinking, *How am I going to tell my husband?*

I told my husband we were pregnant the same day that I found out! I could not keep this a secret. . I was actually quite emotional inside, a ball of nerves! My husband and I were sitting on the couch talking about his day at work. He just returned back to work from being off for our wedding. I remember him asking me "what did you do today?" as I did not return back to work at this time. I began crying instantly and replied "I been trying to figure out how to tell you I am pregnant." The face I saw on my husband's face, I will NEVER forget! He was grinning but with big eyes, staring at me and said "what?" I told him again that I am pregnant. My husband stood up and began walking in the kitchen and I asked what he was doing. He told me "I think I need a beer."

My husband and I were extremely nervous about this pregnancy because it was not planned. Having a child was not at the top of our priority list. Shortly after finding out I was pregnant and we both calmed down from the news, I began bleeding. I miscarriage early in the pregnancy and the doctor had no reason why except "miscarriages are common." We both became very upset over the loss of this baby. Even though the pregnancy was not planned, the loss surprised both of us as our new dreams of a family together were no more. Now I look back and realize how this pregnancy helped our journey to where we are today in the *thoughts* of being parents together.

Our second pregnancy together was planned, but short-lived as the baby passed away in the first trimester. The doctor had scheduled an early ultrasound appointment because of our last miscarriage. At this sonogram appointment we saw a heartbeat! Although the baby was measuring smaller compared to how far along I was in the pregnancy. I was tracking my cycle and knew the approximate day we had conceived.

Shortly after the sonogram appointment, we had another miscarriage. I remember this miscarriage left me feeling very angry and frustrated. I was angry to experience this again and constantly asked why. Why me. I was frustrated and emotionally a wreck because of the loss and the doctor wanting me to try and naturally miscarry on my own. This lasted two weeks before the doctor agreed to a D&C. My uterus did not recognize the baby had passed away, and continued to grow. My thoughts were scattered, and I cried all day and night over this pregnancy loss.

I was scared to miscarry at home. What I would see, and how would I know I had passed the baby's tissue? Then I became very angry when I didn't receive a straight answer from the doctor after the D&C as to what had happened to this pregnancy. The doctor did not follow through on any testing on the baby's tissue (to my knowledge) and said miscarriages are very common and happen all the time, especially because of our age. The doctor explained that after the age of thirty-five, a woman has a 50% chance of miscarrying. That percentage is higher if you have had other miscarriages. This left me feeling hopeless and irate. The doctor gave me no hope and our baby's tissue was thrown away like garbage. We did not know at the time, but we could have requested the baby's tissue, even if we agreed to testing to determine the reason for the loss. Due to the doctor's insensitive nature and understanding, my husband and I decided we'd had enough.

As we researched for a new doctor and completed some blood work, we found out I was pregnant again! So, it appeared I was able to get pregnant easily, which gave me *high* hopes!

This pregnancy was the first where I felt right! It was the first time I could say, "So this is how I am supposed to feel while pregnant!" Nauseous, fatigue, hormonal, cravings!

Then it happened. I was bleeding, with no warning signs, no cramps, no loss of pregnancy symptoms. I simply went to the bathroom and noticed red blood. Panic instantly hit me, tears filled my eyes and I ran out of the bedroom to my husband. Already crying I said, "It's happening again, and showed him blood on a piece of toilet paper." We went to the doctor's office immediately.

We seemed to be sitting in the waiting room forever. I remember looking around the space and seeing pregnant women everywhere, with their hands resting on their bellies as they sat and waited. I reached out to my husband and held his hand for comfort.

When it was our time to be seen by the doctor, we were sent straight for a sonogram. During the sonogram, I knew by the tech's lack of reaction that there was no heartbeat. Plus, I did not see one on the screen. When you live through this situation once, you never forget what to look for on that computer screen. While waiting for the doctor, my husband kept saying over and over "I bet this is normal. Everything will be okay." But when I told him, "No it is not okay, there was no heartbeat on the screen," I could see changes in his face and body language. He went from looking at me, to staring at the floor with his leg bouncing up and down. My husband was trying to prepare himself for the news I have heard too many times: "We could not find a viable heartbeat."

At the time of writing this chapter, that miscarriage happened three weeks ago. I had a D&C completed two weeks ago and we found out the results this week. Our baby had Turner syndrome. This was the first time I found out the sex of my baby. We were pregnant with a girl. My emotions are still all out of sorts. I kept thinking, *I was pregnant with a little girl. A little girl.* I was a little over eight weeks pregnant with her, although we did not find out until eleven weeks that something was wrong. My uterus kept growing, again, not recognizing the loss of the pregnancy for a second time. It is like I am not letting go of the pregnancy. I am not letting go of the baby.

This was my fifth miscarriage. I feel I have had more early pregnancy miscarriages though. I can honestly say anger, more than any other emotion, has guided me through these last few weeks, even the last few years when it comes to this topic. I am angry inside because I do not understand why I cannot have something I feel I 'deserve'. Without trying to sound conceited, I know I am a good person. I am not perfect, and do not want to be perfect, but I want to be a mom. I want to love a child of my own. I want to have a family of my own with my husband. I have wanted this for years, but years ago was not a good time for us. I feel I am hitting a point of disappointment, from my anger, because this is the one thing I have no control over in my life and I am trying so hard to take control of this situation the best way I know how! Back to square one. I wanted answers, and answers are what I received. I needed to understand what Turner syndrome is and whether it will happen again.

From what the OBGYN explained to us, and from what I have researched about the diagnosis, Turner syndrome is also known as gonadal dysgenesis, which is a chromosome disorder for the female gender. Females born with TS only have one X chromosome, which could be an incomplete sex chromosome. If a child is born with TS, it can result in delayed puberty, infertility, and shortness of height, heart defects, and certain learning disabilities. Treatment would involve hormone therapy for life.

I switched doctors this year in my search for answers about my health and reoccurring miscarriages. I switched from a male fertility doctor, to a female OBGYN doctor, hoping she would be more sympathetic to the infertility tests I wanted to request. My last doctor did not feel the need for any blood work, but my new doctor asked why certain testing has not been completed! I remember thinking, *Interesting question!"*

My blood work showed I have two abnormal concerns for blood clot disorders. My protein S free was measuring too low on the scale and my anticardium test was too high. The protein S free measures the level of protein in your blood. Clots can form in your arms and legs, then travel to your lungs. Protein S free is associated with an increased risk of fetal loss and venous thrombosis during pregnancy. It can be hereditary or occur with age. Anticardium is also associated with life-threatening blood clots. The antibody is found in a variety of autoimmune and infectious diseases, such as systemic lupus. This information was provided to me by my doctor and through my own research. I am now on a daily baby aspirin regimen because of the blood clot disorders and if I become pregnant, I have to be placed on a blood thinner injection called Lenox.

Anger and "what-ifs" began to build up in my head with these results!

What if I lost my other babies because of the blood clot disorders?

What if the baby was healthy but my body could not carry him or her because my blood became too thick?

What if I was on medication before this pregnancy, would the results have been the same?

What if our journey to parenthood never materializes?

Those endless "what-ifs" then led to "what then?"

Today I do know that my relationship with my husband is one of the main priorities in my life, with or without children. He is my everything, my partner in life. We are a unit, a team, no matter what, we've got this. My husband and I also still speak about the "what-ifs."

What if we get pregnant again?

What if we decide to adopt?

What if we are not supposed to raise a child and co-parent together?

I am sure there are countless women and couples who understand the way that I feel. How can I explain closure on something that I have no closure to?

However, I can tell you what I have learned about myself so far. I have learned to never stop living, dreaming, praying, and taking care of my own health. I have learned the benefits of gut health for unexplained infertility issues, inflammation within our bodies, MTHFR gene mutation, and vitamins and supplements that we should all be taking—pregnant or not, male and female.

I have learned that there was a relationship missing in my life. I was missing my relationship with God. My relationship with Him has strengthened me on this journey to be a mother and has allowed me to be the best human being possible! I have felt and witnessed His blessings, guidance, love, and relief. The quote below is something I came across, at the right moment. I pray it touches your heart and speaks to you and your journey.

"God is a way-maker. Just know that. The God you serve is a way-maker. He'll make a way to get it done, fix it, shift it, turn it. Even when there doesn't seem to be a way. Get into agreement with God tonight that you're going to serve Him, maintain faith in Him, and wait on Him. Because His blessings are always worth the wait and always right on time."

~ Author Unknown

I believe my babies are happy, healthy, looking down and smiling at their mommy. They each have a front-row seat with Jesus, seeing me day and night, being proud of the woman I strive to be. One day, I will be reunited with my precious angels for eternity. I hope and pray my journey and story finds you peace, support and a better understanding of your own journey.

His Perceptive

As I write and compile this book, there is something I feel that is missed in most pregnancy loss books; the husband's side of the story, or the father explaining his thoughts. It is important to remember that your spouse is also grieving. Your spouse is worried about you; what you are going through, feeling, and thinking. Your husband lost a child too; had his own hopes and dreams ripped from his chest. Dreams that were discussed together because you are building a life together. Here are a few questions and responses that my husband would like to share.

What has been the hardest part on your journey to parenthood with your wife?

It is hard feeling happy, being excited and then feeling upset and helpless during these moments. There have been many ups and downs. The disappointment after feeling hopeful is very difficult. My wife often tells me, "There is nothing you can't fix." This is the one thing I am unable to fix for her----for us.

What could have been done differently by professionals based on our experience?

I wish more professionals would be more helpful. Spending six hours in a hospital room with no help, no answers, and being referred back to your OBGYN is very frustrating. There needs to be more support and understanding during any emergency room visit. I remember both of us feeling more confused and angrier by the time we left the hospital, still with no answers even after a sonogram because no one wanted to deal with this situation. No one wanted to tell us that we lost our child.

What have you learned about yourself in the last few years while trying to have a family with your wife?

You do not think about the struggles you might face when deciding to have a child. You do not often hear about couples having miscarriages, so our journey has not been a typical storybook (journey of getting married, having a home, being financially stable, and then have a family if you choose). I too feel our story is still unknown. Neither of us knows what the future holds.

Final thoughts from Danielle...

To you, the reader, I would like to offer some advice to help you on your journey:

Ask questions and seek help from the right professionals! I did not receive answers until much later in my journey. If something does not seem right to you, find 'your' doctor for help.

Give yourself time to heal and grieve. Find ways to express your feelings. Talk with your spouse or partner, attend a support group, attend counseling, read books, articles and poems that provide understanding and comfort so you do not feel alone.

Pay attention to your health. Learn about gut health and the MTHFR gene mutation. There are a lot of unknown infertility issues and miscarriages caused by poor gut health and having the MTHFR gene mutation. You can request the testing for MTHFR gene mutation through your doctor or through a home testing kit.

Practice gratitude. I am very grateful for my journey to becoming a parent and how my husband and I continue to grow together in our relationship. My husband and I show appreciation and love to one another by actively being in each other's lives. Recognize what you are grateful for within your relationship, your personal life, your health, who you surround yourself with, even your accomplishments. If you are unsure where to begin in recognizing gratitude, start by reflecting on your day, writing at least one thing that you are grateful for, express happiness, thankfulness or even contentment in your life!

If you have a D&C, you may ask for the remains of your baby. The hospital may have you fill out paperwork, but you have the right to your baby's remains, no matter how far along you were in the pregnancy. I did not find this out until recently and I am glad I was made aware of this information to pass it on to my readers.

Psalm 37.7

Be still in the presence of the Lord. Wait patiently for Him to act.

Philippians 4:13

I can do all this through him who gives me strength.

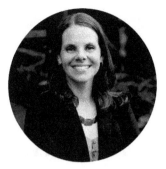

Marcia Allyn

Marcia Allyn is a college professor at Fleming College, with over fourteen years' experience in post-secondary education. Marcia has held positions including publisher, marketing manager, sales representative, and content developer.

As a college professor, Marcia developed curriculum for a course in professional writing. Marcia has a passion for continued learning and tackling new opportunities to drive positive change.

She has written a regular column for the Durham Parents of Multiples newsletter called

Confessions of a Twin Mom.

Outside of work, Marcia has five-year-old twin girls, and loves spending time outside being active and catching up on sleep whenever possible.

Connect with Marcia:
https://www.facebook.com/marciaallyn
https://www.instagram.com/marcia_allyn/
https://twitter.com/marcia_allyn
https://www.linkedin.com/in/marciasiekowski/

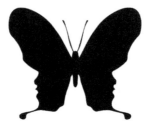

Confessions of a Twin Mom

By Marcia Allyn

It should be the most natural thing in the world: getting pregnant. And it was, for me. Staying pregnant was a whole other story. This is my story.

My husband and I started trying when I was thirty-one. Within a month of going off the pill, I was pregnant. I was elated, walking around the office with a secret smile on my face. Making plans for a nursery. Picking names. My husband had to go out of town for work and I made plans with a friend, let's call her Sara. The night before we were supposed to hang out, I got a horrible headache. I have suffered from migraines all my life, ever since I was a kid, so it was no big deal. I let her know that I would probably have to cancel. I curled up on the couch with an ice pack and some pain killers to ride out the storm. But it just kept getting worse. Eventually, I was writhing in pain with tears streaming down my face. I called Sara and asked if she would take me to the hospital.

Sara had been trying to get pregnant also, without success. As we sat in the waiting room, I told her that I was pregnant. I felt horrible, but I figured she would hear it at some point while I was talking to the nurse or doctor. She said she was happy for me and not to feel guilty at all. What she didn't say was that she suspected my headache meant that something was wrong with the pregnancy.

And because I had always had headaches, I didn't make the connection. I told the doctor so that whatever pain meds he gave me wouldn't affect the fetus and then he sent me home. Sara stayed the night with me and then left in the morning.

When I woke up, I went to the washroom and discovered that I was bleeding. I was immediately terrified. I called Sara and told her that I was going to the walk-in clinic. The doctor there confirmed that it was likely a miscarriage, but that there was nothing I could do. I was devastated. I curled up in bed and cried, sobbing as I thought about this child that wouldn't be born. Even though the doctor said it wasn't my fault, I analyzed everything that I had done over the past couple of months, hoping to find a reason and hoping not to find one at the same time. I felt deflated, physically and emotionally. I told my husband, who was very concerned, especially since he couldn't be there for me. Sara came over and stayed with me again. She suggested we watch movies and eat junk food, trying to distract me from how I felt. When I wanted to talk, she listened. When I cried, she hugged me. She is one of my best friends to this day.

I knew that it wasn't uncommon to miscarry the first time—my own mom had miscarried before she had my sister. It didn't make it any easier though. This new type of headache was caused by the drop in hormones during a miscarriage. So, the problem for me wasn't getting pregnant, it was staying pregnant.

Two months later, I was pregnant again. I felt much more cautious this time around. I began to modify my habits to try and prevent another miscarriage. I eliminated any sort of heavy exercise, started avoiding foods that should be avoided during pregnancy like caffeine, alcohol, deli meat, soft cheese, etc. It wasn't long when I miscarried again.

After the second miscarriage, I went to see my doctor. Since they were within months of each other, even she said that it was unusual to have two so close together. She sent me to a fertility clinic. The doctor I saw (let's call him Dr. D for douchebag), was horrible. He sat across his cluttered desk and said that he didn't think there was an issue at all. He refused to run any tests. Dr. D said, "Come back after you've had a third miscarriage." Douchebag.

One of the most important things I learned from this interaction is to trust your gut. I went back after the third, indignant. He ordered some tests and asked to see my husband, but I still didn't feel as though he was taking me seriously. While I waited for the test results, I had - two more miscarriages. I would feel the heaviness in my uterus, the bloated feeling in my belly, the soreness in my breasts. It felt more comfortable to relax my belly and almost push it out. That there was some resistance when I tried to hold it in. I would analyze every symptom and know in my heart that I was pregnant again, praying that this time would be different.

And then I would miscarry. My hair would fall out and I would have excessive heavy bleeding. I felt inadequate, like somehow, I couldn't do what a woman was meant to do. Like maybe I didn't deserve to be a mother. Like I was somehow a bad person. I would see sixteen-year-olds walking in the mall with their babies and their boyfriends and think, *How can they deserve a baby more than me?* I went to baby showers and put on the fake smile and pretended to be happy for my friends. I was happy for them—I just couldn't hold both sentiments in my heart at the same time, happy and devastated. Devastated won and I faked the rest.

During a follow-up appointment with my own doctor, I expressed my concerns regarding Dr. D. She knew his reputation and was quick to support my request for a second opinion. Sara was happy with her clinic and was now pregnant, so I got a referral. The doctor there was incredibly sympathetic and understanding and ran a comprehensive list of tests. When it was time to go in for the results, she started with my husband—I immediately knew that meant the problem was me.

They told me I have a balanced translocation. Which, in simple terms, means that when I was conceived, two of my chromosomes swapped content. They swapped equal or balanced amounts of content, so it doesn't display as anything for me. However, when my body produces eggs, since it's getting only half of my chromosomes, it doesn't always get the right half. And so, the miscarriages were eggs that weren't genetically viable. This condition is genetic, so it means that it was passed on through the family, but - especially for men- can go undiagnosed since men produce so many sperm at one time, while women only produce one egg each cycle. A large part of me felt relief. At least I knew that I wasn't crazy or imagining the things my body was going through. There was a scientific reason for all of it.

The next step was to see a specialist at Mount Sinai, a geneticist. They explained in much more detail what was happening. The geneticist explained that every month was like a lottery—and eventually, I would get a winning egg. But no one knew when or what percentage of my eggs were good ones. He said that many couples kept trying and sometimes got lucky and when they had enough of trying on their own, they came back to him. What they did is in vitro fertilization, but after fertilizing the eggs they would take a biopsy from each embryo and genetically screen each one. This way they could determine which eggs were viable and only implant the best ones. It was going to be $15,000 to $25,000, depending on how much help I needed. It was terrifying, like literally putting all your eggs in one basket. We decided to keep trying for a while.

I hoped every month would be *the* month. I was getting pregnant roughly every second month, and then before I hit the six-week mark, my body would recognize that it wasn't a viable pregnancy and take care of things. Which is a blessing—mother nature at her finest. But every time my dreams were crushed. Sometimes it would happen so early that I didn't even get a positive pregnancy test. People would say, "Are you sure though, maybe you're not pregnant?" in hopes of easing my distress. Their suggestion crushed me even more and I felt incredibly alone. Just me and my body fighting it out against each other and the world. I kept trying for three years thinking I would win. And finally, I couldn't do it anymore. After seventeen miscarriages, I tapped out.

I wanted to go straight to adoption—I was afraid that after doing IVF we would come out with nothing. After everything I had already been through, it would be crippling to move forward with IVF only to be unsuccessful. At least if we made it through all the screening, adoption would eventually be a sure thing. My husband was less eager to go the adoption route. We had many conversations during the three years trying to get pregnant. By the time I was ready to move on to Plan B, I was so defeated from our failed efforts. My husband said, "Let's just try IVF once, so we know we tried," he said. Because it meant that we were moving forward and I didn't have to keep trying and failing, I reluctantly agreed. As long as we were doing something different from what we had been doing, I was game. And doing IVF taught me another life lesson: don't let fear of failure stop you from trying. And in this case, it paid off.

During this time, my mom and dad, married for forty-three years, split up. I don't need to go into the details of this other than to say that it was incredibly stressful, and I experienced a level of anxiety I hadn't felt before. I couldn't take deep breaths—it felt like an elephant was sitting on my chest. My whole world was rocked. If I thought that my childhood and my family were happy, and I was wrong, how could I consider bringing kids into this world? How could I do any better knowing that my childhood was a farce? We decided to delay IVF for a month or so. I didn't want to sabotage our chances by going into it stressed to the max. I took some time to reconcile everything and decided that even though my parents' marriage was over, my childhood was still a happy one. That's what I focused on instead.

We started IVF after my thirty-fourth birthday. What I will say about this process is that the doctors at Mount Sinai were extraordinary — the right balance of being empathetic and professional. They controlled everything to the smallest detail. I felt I was in very capable hands. Many of the tests and procedures throughout this whole process were painful, invasive, or uncomfortable, but the egg retrieval was the most painful up to that point. It felt like they were scraping my ovaries with a needle. Oh wait, they were. For some reason, the pain medication didn't do a thing to dull the pain. I told them to keep going and just get it done. I produced seventeen eggs that cycle and was extremely happy. Theoretically, once we got a good egg, there was no reason I shouldn't be able to carry to term. They fertilized the eggs and they were incubated for five days. Seven were lost during this time. They biopsied the remaining ten and found that five were defective and/or had my balanced translocation, three others had other chromosomal abnormalities, and two were perfect. That phone call was the moment I had been waiting for, for over three years. I wept tears of grief for the babies that would never come into this world. And tears of joy and hope for the ones that would.

They monitored me closely throughout the pregnancy. After I hit the six-week mark and had my first ultrasound, I knew this time was different. It was real. The pregnancy went fairly smoothly — I was incredibly sick, had horrible heartburn throughout, and went from being vegan to a carnivore almost overnight. But I was happy. I planned for these two little girls, Camryn and Maya, to enter my life. I thought I would stay at home since having two in daycare at the same time would be expensive. I enjoyed every minute, knowing that this would be my one and only pregnancy.

Finally, the day came to have the girls. I was induced after showing some signs of preeclampsia. I was 36.5 weeks pregnant…and HUGE. I stopped weighing myself at 199 lbs. But it was all for the babies and I cooked those buns "real good" (6 lbs 4 oz and 5 lbs 9 oz). I delivered both girls vaginally after twelve hours of active labor. The second one didn't want to come out—she was rather enjoying all the space left after her sister was born. As a result, there were forty long minutes between Maya and Camryn. And as I'm sure happens with many women (having shared my story and heard others), I legitimately thought I was going to die. I started hemorrhaging after Camryn was born and I knew things were going sideways. It was like an episode of Gray's Anatomy—so many doctors and nurses flying around—quietly and calmly doing their thing. I was exhausted beyond anything I had ever experienced before, with vomit on my gown and who knows what on the floor between my legs, my hips aching from the stirrups, hardly able to catch my breath. When I heard Camryn cry, I thought, *If conceiving and giving birth is all I was able to do for them, so be it.* The reality wasn't much better, but I had my babies. That was my next life lesson—you never know what you are capable of until you have no other choice.

We all went home after four days in the hospital. I thought the hard part was over. I was wrong. I started crying on the drive home, thinking, *Now what? What do I do with these babies now?* I was overwhelmed, emotional, still in pain, exhausted.

Over the next several weeks, I slowly started to recover, with a few setbacks. I had some large blood clots and had to go in for a D&C, ending up in the hospital for two nights less than a week after the girls were born, pumping milk to send home. I remember setting my alarm on my phone to wake up and pump. I pumped in the public washroom next to the emergency waiting room. I will never forget the noise the pump made. I literally felt like the life was being sucked out of me, drained and hollow. I pumped for the girls for a month and then got mastitis, an infection in the breast caused by a blocked milk duct. It felt like the most horrible flu ever. My body ached, I had a fever, and all my energy was completely consumed in fighting the infection. When I finally sought medical help, the doctor at the walk-in clinic gave me two different antibiotics and warned me that if it didn't get better within twenty-four hours, I was to go to the emergency room. My breast was at a critical point where it might explode in order to get rid of the infection. I tapped out again.

I weaned myself off of pumping while I was on the antibiotics so that I wouldn't get mastitis again. Switching to formula meant that I didn't have to get up and pump every three to four hours and it meant that anyone could feed the girls, so I finally got some uninterrupted sleep. That first eight-hour sleep was magical. It definitely made a huge difference in my recovery. The decision to stop pumping (while controversial to some) allowed me to keep it together, at least until the girls started showing signs of acid reflux. Then every feeding became a nightmare. And I broke.

My mom came in one morning and I was sitting there with a pile of used tissue crumpled on the coffee table, tears streaming down my face. All I had eaten were some oatmeal cookies she made the day before. I couldn't stop crying. I felt like the worst mom in the world. I couldn't even feed my own babies. They would scream from the pain of the acid reflux and if I didn't feed and burp them just right, they would projectile vomit and I would have to start all over again. Trying to do this for one baby while the other one is crying to be fed, it was all too much.

From that day on, until the reflux was under control with medication, I had help every day. Our families were amazing. My mom encouraged me to go to the doctor after finding me that morning and my doctor started me on medication for post-partum depression. Another life lesson: ask for help and accept the help that's given. I was willing to accept any help being offered if it would help me to be a better mom for my girls.

I am still on medication to this day. I don't think you can ever truly recover from PPMD (post-partum mood disorders). Just like with infertility, as soon as I started talking about it, I found so many others who struggled as well. I found comfort in not being alone. I found a tribe of women who would never judge me and who would always be there to help. Some of my best friends are present in my life because of the struggles we went through together. For me, this was harder than any part of the infertility process. It wasn't just crying all day. It wasn't just a lack of attachment to my babies. It was like a dark sleeping monster inside me had awakened. I didn't know who I was anymore. I went from being indifferent and zombie-like to being angry at the drop of a hat. I would get so frustrated that I had to walk away from the babies. I felt the overwhelming urge to bite their cheeks or walk out the front door and never come back. It brought on a whole other level of guilt— maybe I wasn't meant to have children after all. Maybe I had infertility to prevent this from happening. Maybe they would be better off with another mom. I knew I needed more help.

In addition to the medication, monitored closely by my family doctor, I went through a cognitive behavioral therapy program specifically for PPMD. My social worker was kind, real, non-judgemental, and amazingly helpful to me. I realized that between the miscarriages, the fertility treatment, and the twin pregnancy, I was probably always going to get PPMD of some kind. It was a hormonal recipe for disaster. During this time, I also went back to work—that was monumental for my mental health. Having time away from the girls allowed me to miss them and to come home eager to see them. It allowed me to love them, finally, in the way that I wanted to from the beginning. I have learned more about myself since I had my girls than I have my whole life up until then. I learned to work with myself instead of against myself. I've learned to listen to myself in ways I never had before. I know now that I have to be at my best as a person in order to be at my best as a mom. And, maybe most importantly, I've learned that the best things in life are worth the struggle.

It's helped me to know that everyone has their own story. You can't know what a person has struggled with until you talk to them. Being a mom isn't easy, but I will never judge another parent (or person for that matter). Sharing my story has been therapeutic for me, but also helped others to open up. I try to encourage anyone who's willing to share their story as well, to help support each other and also to end the stigma regarding infertility, miscarriage, stillbirth, infant loss, postpartum mood disorders, and any other stigma. Let's share our grief instead of keeping silent, support each other to promote healing, and celebrate the hope we have in our hearts.

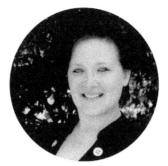

Ashlee Boice

Ashlee Brianna resides in New Castle Pennsylvania and is currently working in the insurance Industry. She is a married mother of four, with their most recent addition coming through kinship adoption in the summer of 2017. When she is not cheering her little ones from the sports stands, she is providing full-time care for her disabled father and working to finish her degree in business administration from Slippery Rock University.

Ashlee is currently enjoying the process of redesigning and remodeling her hundred-year-old fixer upper home and she is hoping the passion will lead to an opportunity to start her own design business in the future.

Connect with Ashlee:
https://www.facebook.com/ashlee.boice
https://www.instagram.com/boiceashlee/

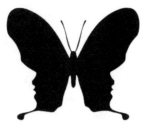

Angel Baby

By Ashlee Boice

July 10th, 2007 was the day I mustered the courage to take the test. At barely twenty-one years old, I was already a young unmarried mother to a ten-month-old daughter.

What if it's positive? Could we handle another child so soon? Another unplanned pregnancy, how will my mom feel? Our relationship has been a bit rocky. Can we handle this? So many questions within a three-minute waiting period. If I told you I actually remembered taking the test for my second child, I would be lying. I remember testing for my first daughter, and I remember the tests for the third and fourth. I can picture each of them, but not the test for my second child. I remember every thought and fear, but I can't visually remember taking the test. Why? Trauma response? Maybe.

Positive! I don't remember telling anyone, but they knew! Trauma response? I remember in great detail every other child's announcement. Why can't I break through? They say the mind will patch trauma with holes in your memory.

A few days after testing, I remember my cousin, Tommy, sharing the news with me that he and his girlfriend were also expecting. Calculations placed us both expecting in March 2008! *Wow! How cool is this going to be? How cool would it be for them to share the same birthday?* I thought.

When I started to become excited about having another child, our world became rocky. I started bleeding. Even at the tender age of twenty-one, I knew blood was a scary sign of trouble. In a panic, we hoped a trip to the emergency room would ease our fears.

They took me back for an ultrasound scan, and a very small spot on the screen showed a healthy heartbeat at roughly six-week gestation. I was told to take it easy and to schedule an appointment with my doctor for follow up care.

A week later, I went to my appointment. Up to this point, the bleeding was light but consistent. Further discussion with my doctor proved informative. He advised that bleeding in early pregnancy can actually be common, as it could just be old blood, and that as long as the consistency was light and the color remained brown, we were okay. Red blood was the sign of real trouble and if I saw any I was to call him immediately.

Throughout the next two weeks, my stress levels were elevated due to hardships in my relationship and finances, but no alarming signs that me and baby were in any trouble. I even continued to work at a normal pace.

On August 7, 2007, I was scheduled to work a full eight-hour shift at my job. I worked as a shift manager at a local McDonald's at the time, which required long hours on my feet with little to no breaks. During this particular shift, I noticed I wasn't feeling very well. I was very tired and weak. Continuing on, I contributed the feelings to early pregnancy symptoms. Until I felt it. A sharp pain and the feeling of a gush of blood.

I rushed to the restroom to check, and there it was, a large bright red clot of blood. "Bright red means bad," I yelled as I began to cry. We were in trouble. I called Doctor Joe and explained what I discovered. He advised me to head straight to the hospital to be checked out. I cleaned up the best I could and called my then partner, Shawn, to let him know that something was wrong.

At the time, he and my cousin, Tommy, worked together at a construction company and were on their way home for the day. Instead, they headed to Ellwood City Hospital, as I drove myself to meet them there.

After we got there, the three of us waited for what felt like forever to be called back for the scan. I lay on the bed, Shawn sat in the chair right beside me, and Tommy sat in a chair in the corner behind him. As the technician began the scan, I suddenly felt a sense of dread, the room was eerily quiet, and the technician's energy changed. She continued the scan and I saw what appeared to be our baby on the screen, and for a split second, I had a glimmer of hope. Until the technician turned to us and said, "I'm sorry, I can't find the heartbeat." I was in shock! My heart raced and tears streamed down my face. I looked over at Shawn, who also looked to be in shock, searching for a way to process the news. But then I looked at Tommy, and for some reason, at that moment, when I saw this man crying for us and our baby, it hit me hard like a ton of bricks. I had up, until that day, only saw that man cry one time in my life—the day his dad passed away. For some reason his tears made it real.

After the scan, the technician told us Doctor Joe would be waiting for us downstairs. His office was in the basement area of the hospital at the time. On the way to his office, the devastation really began to hit me. Was this because I focused on not being ready? Did I bring negative energy into my space and cause this to happen? Were my bad thoughts and questions in the beginning the reason for this? What did I do wrong? As the nurse walked us back to his office, my legs got weak and I felt sick to my stomach.

Shawn and I were seated in the doctor's personal office, while Tommy waited in the waiting room.

The doctor came in and began explaining that our baby was still there, but that no heartbeat was detected during the scan. He offered to schedule another scan the following Monday to check again, but explained that if a heartbeat was still not detected, a dilation and curettage, commonly referred to as a D&C, would be required if the baby was still there.

So, we scheduled and went home for the weekend to collect our thoughts and emotions. We felt everything from despair to anger during that long weekend. Monday morning came and I found myself back on the scan table to learn the final fate of our baby.

No heartbeat.

I had the procedure and was sent home with instructions to refrain from attempting to "try again" for at least one regular cycle.

Try again? That weighed heavy for me. This was an unplanned pregnancy, but now I felt so empty. Try again? Did we want that? There were so many concerns and fears when we found out about our angel baby. For weeks I fought the urge to act out of my grief. I didn't want to "try again" for the sole purpose of filling the void I carried every day.

Somehow, this experience seemed to bring Shawn and I closer together. What was a rocky relationship began to find its foundation again, and we focused on rebuilding the following six weeks.

In October, Shawn asked me what I was feeling and what I wanted to do going forward. I confided in him that I wanted to have my children close in age, but I feared the only reason we would try again was to simply attempt to fill the void we were experiencing. Further discussion brought us to the decision to move forward and try again, and in November 2007, we experienced the joy again of a positive pregnancy test.

However, just two weeks later, the bleeding returned. It started out brown. Due to my history, my doctor decided to monitor us much more closely, and a scan was performed. Everything appeared normal and our baby had a strong heartbeat. Music to my ears!

In December 2007, I received a devastating call. My Uncle Jim had passed of a massive heartache the night before. This was the first really close loss that I had experienced up to that point with the generation older than mine. He was a wonderful father figure to me when mine skipped out. Even from several states away, he had more influence than most.

The services were scheduled on December just a few days after Christmas in Indiana, a six-hour drive from home. I called my doctors due to the current complications because I wanted approval to travel. He agreed but I had to promise that if anything abnormal happened I would call him immediately, regardless of the distance between us. On, Shawn's birthday, we packed up and the whole family caravanned to Fort Wayne, Indiana to be with each other at a difficult time.

During the scheduled viewing the night before the services, a very familiar feeling washed over me and I rushed to the restroom in a panic. There it was, bright red! I immediately broke down and cried. *Not again. I can't handle this again.*

Shawn again rushed me to the emergency room, only this time I was two states away from my doctor, who was powerless to help me. Again, I waited for what felt like forever to be taken back to the scan room. It was really stressful being in a strange hospital, with strangers in charge of our care this time, to learn the fate of our baby.

This time, as I lay on the table in a silent room, a heartbeat fluttered across the speakers! It was there and it was strong! I began crying tears of joy! In my mind, nothing anyone could say would matter, because I heard the heartbeat with my own ears. However, not all the news was good. Yes, our baby was still with us and it had a strong heartbeat, but we were in serious trouble.

Placental abruption, a condition where the placenta separates from the uterus, can be a serious condition and leads to a high rate of miscarriages—and we had a tear. The doctors advised me that we had an 80% chance of losing our baby, and that strict bedrest was necessary.

After returning home, I went in to see Doctor Joe. Of course, bedrest was ordered, and he repeated the statistical chances of another miscarriage in these situations. Prepared, but not ready to give up, I followed strict orders, and each time they found a strong heartbeat on the doppler during my appointments.

During our twenty-week scan, we learned that the baby was a girl and she was growing great and looked healthy, but one piece of news brought more tears of joy. The tear was gone, it had healed, and we were stronger than ever.

The remainder of our pregnancy was uneventful. Shawna, named for her daddy, was due to join us on August 8, 2008. I craved snickers and lucky charms and loved everything in the color hot pink. I usually hate pink!

Then, on July 7, 2008, fear hit us again when we were rushed to the hospital with what I assumed was false labor pains. It turned out to be real labor pains and the doctor announced that I was four centimeters at thirty-five weeks. We were not ready! She had another month to grow first.

To keep her from delivering early, the doctors felt it was safest to intervene and stop our labor. Armed with medicine and orders of strict bedrest, yet again, we were released with the hope that the intervention would keep us pregnant for at least another week.

Just two days later, on July 9th, the contractions began again, and a call to Doctor Joe had us rushing back into the hospital again. This time it was too late to intervene. I was far along—six centimeters on arrival.

Our birth plan for Shawna was to attempt a VBAC or vaginal birth after C-section. Due to the risks involved, a required OR team was placed on stand-by. Also due to her premature gestation, a life-flight team was required to be on stand-by due to the small hospital not being equipped with a NICU unit.

After just six hours of active labor, Shawna Brianne was born at 2:25 am on July 10, 2008, via a successful VBAC delivery. She was a perfectly healthy 6 lbs 6 oz and needed no additional support after birth.

Our rainbow after the storm, our incredible story of loss, love, and hope.

On August 7, 2010, on the third anniversary of the loss of our daughter, we honored her and each other by exchanging our wedding vows and, today our rainbow baby, Shawna, is eleven years old and we were blessed with a son three years later. We have also walked the journey of adoption with our youngest daughter, who was born in 2017. We will never forget our angel baby. We honor her through memories every day, and talk about her often with our children, because she is part of their sibling circle. Even if she is not present, her story will live on through us.

If I could pass any advice to you it would be lean on your support system. My family is a huge part of how I get through troubling times in my life. Find your support and lean on them. Remember you are stronger than you believe. When you think you can't handle anymore, you somehow will find the strength to keep going. And last but not least, your spouse is your partner in all of this, remember you are not alone in your journey. Use this time to connect on a deeper level with them.

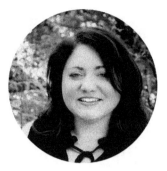

Summer Corbin

Summer is an educator with twenty years' experience in public and charter schools. She has a dual Bachelor's Degree in Elementary and Special Education from Geneva College as well as graduate work in creative writing at the University of Tampa.

As a trauma survivor, she understands how disclosure and vulnerability can be difficult, but also a starting point for healing and creativity.

Summer is an avid reader, traveler, and amateur genealogist. She is an introvert but believes strongly that sharing your story can be a catalyst for healing—both for herself and others. She considers herself a fan of authors and researchers Brene Brown and Kay Redfield Jamison, and loves all topics related to mental health.

Connect with Summer:
https://www.facebook.com/summer.corbin.5
www.OnceUponATimeDear.com

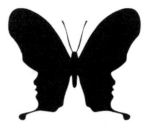

Getting Back Up

By *Summer Corbin*

I had warned Jason prior to the wedding that I did not want him smashing the cake in my face ruining my makeup. It was supposed to be stifling hot 85 degrees and humid and sugar-coated skin in that heat would only make me uncomfortable. At the moment though, when I saw the laughter in his brown eyes, I knew what was coming! Jason was a jokester. Pre-emptively, though, I reached up and swiped my raspberry filled vanilla slice across his forehead. In less than a second came the revengeful full thrust of his entire slice into my powdered nose and down I went in a balloon of ruffles and lace. There was a collective gasp from the friends and family who had come out to support us on this beautiful Saturday afternoon and then a ruckus of laughter as Jason and my horrified wedding planner pulled me to my feet.

Today, however, was a cold blistering January day as I sat on the floor staring at the First Response pregnancy test in my shaky hand. This time, Jason was nowhere around to pull me back to my feet. There it was: *pregnant*. I blinked in disbelief and thought about the dozens of negative pregnancy tests tossed in the trash over the last two years.

Flushed and unsteady, I reached for my iPhone. I placed the plastic test on the floor and centered it within the frame of my camera, and with some reservations

I found 'Mom' in my contact's list and pressed send.

Twenty minutes later, Mom still had not responded. I checked 'read receipts' repeatedly. *She never checks her phone dammit*, I thought, glancing up at the box of pregnancy tests on the dresser. There was one left.

My phone vibrated.

Mom: Are you *sure?*

Annoyed, I put the phone down on the bed without responding. I grabbed the First Response box off the dresser.

Chugging a Gatorade, I made my way back into the bathroom.

Three minutes. *I'm not gonna watch it*, I thought. *I'm not gonna watch it. I'm not gonna watch* it.

I stood frozen in front of the sink: *Not pregnant.*

Mom picked up on the first ring. "I'm not pregnant. I took another test." I sobbed into the phone and shook in the silence that followed.

"Summer, you don't know," she said. "You had one test that was positive! I think you need to go to the doctor and get a blood test."

Two years prior, I laid across our queen bed and shoved my list of names across the bedsheet to Jason, who was concentrating on surfing Netflix. Jason was a teddy bear of a guy and I snuggled up next to him and tapped the list again. "You're okay with another child?" I asked him. I had three awesome stepchildren from my relationship with Jason, but I dearly longed for a child with him.

Not waiting for an answer, I asked, "What's your name for a boy?" He smiled at me but hesitated.

"You're okay with another child, right?"

"Sure. I think Zeke Zellem has a ring to it." He smiled gingerly.

"And if I should ever have a girl, you're okay with me choosing the name?" He grabbed my list off the bed.

He grinned. "You only have one name on this list!"

"That's because I've known for over a decade my name for a girl: Valerie Victoria Kaye Zellem."

He cocked his head slightly with a lighthearted smile. "So, you knew ten years ago that you would be a 'Zellem'? Coyly, I kissed his cheek. "No silly, Valerie and Kaye to honor my doctors and Victoria to honor my mother."

"Do you think that your medications will impact your ability to get pregnant? Is it safe I mean?" I looked at Jason. His concern was not lost on me. I'd had numerous conversations with my psychiatrist Dr. Kaye, and we had decided to try alternative medications and she was keeping me on the lowest doses I could take for bipolar disorder. There were other things, besides medications, that I had to think through and take into consideration. The biggest of these being sleep deprivation after a baby is born and the possibility that I could find myself in a depressive state or a manic episode due to hormonal changes that come with pregnancy and childbirth.

"I know the risks baby, but it's worth it to me to be a mother." I had been working with my doctors—Dr. Kaye as well as my therapist, Val, for over ten years. I trusted them implicitly and they had both seen me through the highs and lows of my manic-depressive illness. Their guidance over the years had helped enable me to stay stable and well. With their support, I was going forward with our plans to try to get pregnant.

Jason answered the phone on the third ring. "I have to go to the hospital for a pregnancy test. I have an appointment tomorrow. Can you go with me?" Jason worked long hours and I know he heard my disappointment when he told me he could not. I had long been wondering if Jason truly wanted a child with me. He seemed to be quieter about it, and appeared to have reservations he wouldn't say out loud.

I sat alone in the Beaver Valley Medical Center, clutching my iPhone and updating my mother: They had me take a standard urine-pregnancy test. The reading indicated I was pregnant. I now sat waiting to be called in for the blood test. This would be it… the moment. We had been trying for two years. *I am thirty-nine years old and have been trying for two years. That's not a long time compared to some women, but I am pushing forty and running out of time!*

"Mrs. Zellem?" Shaking, I followed a woman who looked to be in her twenties into the lab room, and sat down in the pleather chair. "They usually use the butterfly technique on me because I have shallow veins," I told her. She smiled, "Thanks for telling me!" The whole process was fast, and I found myself sitting back in the waiting room awaiting the results.

I sat there, bargaining with God. *Please let me be pregnant. Please let me be pregnant.* I made silent deals with Him but there was silence in response to my prayers.

It seemed like an hour passed before I was called into the room again with the doctor. "I'm sorry", she began. My heart sank and I didn't feel steady even sitting. "The hCG levels were present, but not high enough to produce a positive result."

"What does that mean?" I asked her. "It's the loss of a pregnancy prior to the twentieth week. I know this is painful and I am sorry."

"But my period is late, and the pregnancy tests that were positive!"

She nodded empathetically. "Your period should come within a few days. Again, I'm sorry. The good news is that you *can* get pregnant, though"

I made my way numb out into the cold, windy, parking lot. I repeated to myself over and over, "I was pregnant. I *was* pregnant."

I climbed up into my Hyundai SUV and began sobbing hysterically. For a little while, I was a mother… I sat weeping for the child I would never hold.

I had two chemical pregnancies in the course of three years. I kept the second one to myself from the start because I was so fearful of going through the pain and disappointment that can come with sharing. In my mind, Valerie Victoria Kaye Zellem and Zeke Zellem are waiting for me in heaven, where I'll get to meet them someday. I think naming my unborn children has helped me process the pain.

I'll never know if my medications or my age affected my ability to carry a healthy embryo. My doctor was careful about selecting medications based on research with pregnancy… but bipolar disorder must be treated properly with medication. Whether or not to take medication wasn't a debate for me.

Sadly, our marriage became rocky in 2018, shortly after Jason told me he did not want a child with me. Jason filed for divorce in July of 2019. I was forty-two, divorcing, and a child was no longer an immediate possibility. I was forced at this point to look sincerely at where I was in life and what I could change and what I could not.

Throughout my struggles with infertility, I vacillated between denial and acceptance. That's because acceptance of anything painful is a process that comes in stages. I had so many fears revolving around not being whole or good enough if I wasn't a mother. Often, I would ruminate about how my parents might be feeling about not having any grandchildren and it would devastate me.

In addition to that, because of my illness, I had always felt marginalized and rejected. Much of these feelings of shame stemmed from my insistence on hiding who I was. My fear of being an outsider to society was so strong that I kept my diagnosis to myself and even denied, to myself and others, that I had an illness. That all changed whenever I began to speak candidly about my life, first to my family, and then to friends… and even some acquaintances.

Something that helped me face my fears and console me was the practice of radical acceptance—a mindfulness technique that I learned in psychotherapy. Radical acceptance revolves around accepting that you are your emotions, your circumstances, your past, and your pain. Failure to accept these things delays healing. Accepting pain and allowing yourself time to process it allows you to grow and problem solve. It lets you release what you have no control over and lets us focus on the control that we do have.

The first step in implementing radical acceptance is to notice that you are resisting reality. You have to be able to admit to yourself that some things are out of your control and recognize how your response to it affects your thoughts and feelings. Acknowledging this is difficult but it is the first step towards healing. I struggled with this for the longest time, but healing and peace came from my being able to recognize I was resisting my reality.

The second step is to comfort that part of yourself that hurts. It helps to develop coping skills to deal with your feelings. Accepting reality is difficult when life is painful. However, validating your feelings about your sense of loss is important and part of the journey towards radical acceptance. Validating your emotions can be a simple as saying to yourself, "I'm terribly sad that things are not the way I hoped they would be and it's ok to feel this for now."

The third step is to turn your mind toward acceptance…again, and again. You can physically do this by speaking out loud the serenity prayer. You could also sit down and create a gratitude list for your life's blessings. This will help you let go of the ideas about how you "should be" and accept the way you are and the reality that you are living.

As a Christian, I found the following verse to be a cornerstone for radical acceptance and for my healing: Jeremiah 29:11 "For I know the plans I have for you," declares the Lord. "Plans to prosper you and not to harm you. Plans to give you a hope, and a future." Reading this, my focus began to change from what I will not be to *who I am* and *what I am called to do in this world.*

I have not 'arrived' anywhere other than acceptance. I have an honorary niece, Ella, and an honorary nephew Tobias, born to a dear friend… who mean the world to me and whom I can now be present for in a way that I struggled to be when I could not accept my circumstances regarding having children.

In 2019, in the midst of divorce, and sadness over my not being a mother, I picked myself back up off the floor. I started by looking around for the things that I *am* grateful for and the things that make my life worthwhile *right now.* My family, my church, my friends, my work, and even my readers are all reasons to get up every morning, put my feet on the ground and give it my all. That is my hope for any reader whom this story resonates with: that you will count every blessing and every morning you will get up and give it your all.

Learning that happiness does not have to be fulfillment of your personal desires has been a big step forward for me to be able to move on toward other personal goals. Happiness can be a choice right now, where you are in your present situation, and I think that is what God calls us to do.

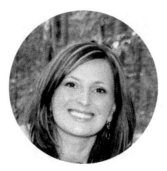

Joyce Foley

Joyce Foley is a long-time resident of Chardon, Ohio, where she raises her five rambunctious boys.

Joyce has always had a passion in caring for others and earned her nursing degree just out of high school. As she built a family of her own, she continued her studies earning her bachelors and then going on to complete her Masters in Nursing as a pediatric nurse practitioner.

Between 2017- 2019, Joyce found herself the patient in a battle with bone cancer. Her unfailing faith and strong support system guided her through as she beat the disease. In the process, she became an amputee. Mobility has been challenging but she enjoys getting out and embracing fun with her children whenever she can.

Connect with Joyce:
Foleyfive831@gmail.com
https://www.facebook.com/joycefoley1

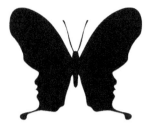

Forever in My Heart

By Joyce Foley

Ever since I can remember, I have dreamed of being a mother. I imagined two boys and two girls, and had names already picked out since I was young. Never could I have realized where this wild journey of motherhood would take me. Each and every one of my pregnancies has its own story, but I am here to share one that broke me down and lifted me back up in ways I could not have imagined.

At the age of twenty-four, I developed severe abdominal pain and I was sent to the emergency room for suspected appendicitis. It was there that I had a scan which revealed a uterine deformity and a single kidney. I could not believe that I had come this far in life not knowing these crucial things about myself. Then again, I found myself lucky that I had never experienced any secondary complications. I began researching everything I could on this anomaly, only to worry myself more. You never think that it is going to be you that has a problem when it comes to having a child. You never think that you will be the one facing troubling issues in life.

I was sent to see a specialist and advised to undergo diagnostic testing to assure that my fallopian tubes were open, as this could affect my ability to conceive. Following these tests, I was told I had two completely separate uteri, each with their own single ovary. With this anomaly, the chances of me conceiving or carrying a fetus to term would be unlikely. If I did conceive, I was advised that I would never be able to deliver naturally as my anatomy was so unusual that it would not allow a natural course. My mind swirled with emotions. I felt like I had been punched in the stomach. *Could this really be happening to me?* I was newly married and had no plans to have a baby for a few years, but the fear of infertility changed my plans drastically. I consulted more than one obstetrician, making sure that I had the right information at my fingertips. My husband and I took the plunge, deciding that we needed to start trying now rather than wait and have any further issues.

To my surprise, I became pregnant later that year. Due to my unusual condition, I was considered high-risk and had to see a specialty obstetrician. For this, I was thankful as I had frequent ultrasound scans to assure my baby was developing appropriately.

My first pregnancy was filled with anxiety and fear of the unknown. I questioned every little ache or pain that did not feel right. I wish now that I could go back and have thoroughly enjoyed the experience.

As it turns out, that pregnancy was relatively uneventful until the third trimester, when I began to have elevated blood pressure, requiring more tests and visits to the hospital. It persisted to the point I required an emergency C-section at thirty-six weeks. All those worries washed away as soon as I held my perfect, healthy son.

My second pregnancy was very similar, as was my third… both ending in early C-sections related to elevated blood pressure. It felt blessed to have beat all the odds that were stacked against me.

After three pregnancies with successful deliveries, it felt as though my family was complete. I now had three young boys who looked up to me, calling me "mommy." I may not have had the two boys and two girls that I had imagined, but my dreams had been answered. I decided it was time to refocus myself on my career, where I had left off before having my first child.

I pursued my master's degree while working full-time and raising my boys. Everyone around me felt I was unreasonable for taking on so much, but I was determined as always to reach my goals. During my third and last year of graduate school an urge to have just one more baby came over me. As though I needed one more to join my rambunctious crew. The previous three years had flown by and I missed having an infant in my arms. This was not a decision that came lightly with my known risks, and I consulted my obstetrician to assure I was being safe. The thought sounded selfish, and maybe it was, though not one I would ever regret.

It was a bit more of a struggle to conceive this time around. In the end, if it was meant to be it would be. There was no pressure or ovulation tracking, not like before. Several months later, my prayers were answered, we were expecting! I excitedly awaited my first appointment and received my first ultrasound around six weeks. The obstetrician was always aware to scan each uterus to be sure that there was not a pregnancy in both sides. At that first visit, only one baby was seen in my right uterus. Two weeks later, my ultrasound revealed a second pregnancy in my left uterus. This was not the news I was expecting, and I was told that things were about to get a lot more difficult for me. With my condition, this created a dangerous scenario. I was told the chances of sustaining both babies to term would be very slim. Although worried, I was determined to beat the odds as I had three times before.

I began planning for these two precious little ones. The thought that they would share such a special bond touched me deeply. Growing from a family of five to a family of seven would be tough but it would be just one more adventure I would learn to navigate.

During each of my appointments, I enjoyed watching my babies grow strong, and my dreams for them were endless. At sixteen weeks I learned that we were expecting two more boys... *oh boy!*

At around twenty weeks, I began having left-sided back pain that became increasingly worse. I initially blew this off, blaming it on my body adjusting to the pregnancy. As the pain escalated, I noticed blood in my urine and asked to be seen by my doctor. I had an ultrasound of my kidney and found that I had developed stones. Kidney stones are extremely painful, though worse when you only have one kidney and there is blockage creating severe lower back spasms. I began to have complications related to the stones. I was in and out of the hospital receiving a good amount of pain medication. I was afraid of the effects this would have on my babies but was assured that the doses were safe. There were no interventions I could undergo for the stones while I was pregnant due to the risks to my single kidney. The best-case scenario would be passing the stones on my own. Unfortunately, that never happened. I quickly learned that standing up continuously during the day and lying in a recliner on my right side at night were the only things that could help me be the least bit comfortable. I tried to avoid the pain medication as much as I could, though it was often unbearable.

When I went in for my twenty-four-week appointment, I felt relatively well. I remember the ultrasound technician and I had an upbeat conversation just before she put the gel on my belly. I could never have prepared myself for what was coming next.

She first scanned my right uterus as they always had, and I quickly knew something was very wrong by the concerned look on her face. Without skipping a beat, she jumped to the left uterus, which showed a very wiggly baby. I froze, and time seemed to stand still before she shared her concerns and went for the obstetrician to review. It was then that I learned that my baby in my right uterus had no heartbeat. I felt as though I was choking and could not catch my breath. My life as I had imagined it immediately shattered. Nothing about this situation felt real and I felt this could not possibly be happening to me. I somehow managed to pull myself together as several questions came to mind. Were they really sure that my baby had passed away? I demanded that they check again, and I stared at the screen, endlessly waiting for a glimmer of hope that never came. A sense of dread came over me as I anxiously asked if I had I killed my baby by taking all those pain medications. I was told that they could not know for sure the effects the medications might have had. The rational me knew that this was not my fault, but I needed to place the blame somewhere, and in those moments, it was on myself. I was told that this was considered a late-term loss as my baby passed some time in the second trimester. With two completely separate uteri, I was assured that the death of this twin would not affect the other. There were risks for infection carrying a deceased baby and I would have to be monitored even more closely than before. The hope was to get me as close to term as we could before delivering.

I worried what would become of my deceased baby. Not knowing the exact timing of fetal demise made it hard to determine. I was told that my body could start to break down the tissues and reabsorb the tissue, or the fetus could slowly get smaller as the fluids would reabsorb. The thought of carrying my deceased baby with these awful things happening to him sickened and overwhelmed me. How could I possibly go through the rest of my pregnancy carrying a healthy baby while slowly losing the other? I was told that situations like this happened all the time and the body has a way of naturally "dealing" with it. I was dismissed by the doctors who said it was probably for the best as the chances of me carrying both of the boys with my uterine anomaly would have been too risky anyways. It was almost as though they were relieved that they would not have to deal with any complications in the end. This caused me so much anger and frustration, it is something that stayed with me for a very long time.

As I left my appointment, I was not sure how I would possibly break the news to my other boys or my husband. I tried to hold back, but found myself breaking down and sharing everything as soon as I got home. I thought my husband would have been supportive, though he too said that it was probably for the best. He could not fathom the thought of handling two more children. He was so unsympathetic in those moments. This hurt me in ways I could not explain.

Unfortunately, it is something that we would never be able to put behind us. As I tried to wrap my head around what everyone was telling me, I felt like I was slowly dying inside. I had to have frequent ultrasounds, and eventually, I stopped looking at the monitor as I did not want to see what had become of my baby boy. They did share that he was slowly getting smaller as the doctors had speculated. As the fetus in my left uterus grew stronger each day, the other slowly disappeared. My thoughts consumed me as I walked around every day knowing that the baby I had hoped for and dreamed about was gone. Emotionally, this is one of the hardest issues I had ever faced. I became extremely depressed as I worried about the health of the surviving twin.

I spent every day grieving my loss, blaming myself. I again felt selfish in my thoughts… *I should be happy to still have one healthy baby.* At least that is what friends kept telling me. I do not know why we say things like that to people in our lives, and we are all guilty of it. Unless you have gone through something similar it is hard to fully understand or to be able to give reasonable advice. I no longer wanted to hear what anybody around me had to say and I stopped telling others, especially my family, what I was going through. I did not want their thoughts on the situation as I continuously felt brushed off. I did not want anybody telling me how blessed I was to have three healthy children. I *was* blessed, but that did not take away the heartache and devastation I felt inside, because I did not want just one, I wanted *both* of my babies.

I struggled to get through my days and to take care of myself and my family, but I faithfully went to every appointment to make sure that my baby was thriving. If I had to endure the loss of him too, I was not sure how I would make it through. The kidney stones continued to complicate the pregnancy and I chose to bear through the discomfort rather than take anything else that could potentially harm my baby.

I remember making it to thirty-six weeks and feeling that was such a feat. I had never made it beyond that in the past. I knew we were now in the home stretch and I could not wait for the day my baby would be in my arms. However, the fear of losing him still consumed my every thought.

The stones eventually caused a blockage and began to swell significantly. It was incredibly uncomfortable, and I struggled physically. Through this, I continued my studies and my full-time job. I needed these things to occupy my mind, to help me run from my depression and anxiety. I thought about seeking psychological help but again feared more medications. That was something that I would seek out later.

A C-section was scheduled for thirty-eight weeks. The countdown to that date dragged on. The morning I entered the hospital for surgery I was again completely and utterly overwhelmed with hope and grief. I did not know what to expect moving forward, and for the first time found myself consoled by another, a labor and delivery nurse who was seasoned and had seen it all. The delivery was complicated by extremely low blood pressure and I became very ill in the operating room. Through the haze I heard the nurses talking, exclaiming how cute my little one was and

Compiled by Danielle Lynn

commenting on his dimpled chin. I remember thinking, *He's finally here, he's alive and he's all mine.* The moment I was well enough, I embraced him and I never wanted to let him go. I had felt these emotions following the delivery of my other children, but not on this level.

He was perfect in every way. I stared at him and imagined having another just like him. I felt such a loss for my boy, for the twin he would never meet. Over the next few days, my body began to naturally bleed, as it does following any pregnancy, though this time I also passed what was left of my deceased child. No words can explain what that does to someone, especially a mother. I found myself sitting in the bathroom endlessly and grieving his loss all over again.

Somehow, my newest little one would get me through that hard time. Without him, I would have never come back from the depths of despair. My other children were wonderful and embraced him. We spent every minute we could together, and the guilt still came as I thought about the little one I would never mother. But with time, the guilt faded.

Through all of this, the support I had was minimal from those I expected it from the most. After some time, I knew I needed to seek professional help. Adding postpartum hormones on top of an already depressed and anxious mother is a recipe for disaster. I did not care about the stigma around it or what anybody else thought, but I knew that I could not be the mother I wanted to be without seeking professional help.

I found a way to memorialize my baby by wearing a chain around my neck with all of my children's names and a large circle with footsteps stating 'forever in my heart'. He was real and he was mine. He made me realize my worth as a mother. I never did name him, though I now wish I had. Maybe giving him a name would have helped make my dream more of a reality. At the time, I did not want that to be my primary focus. If I gave him a name and talked about him, I would have to share his story over and over again. At that time, it was not something that I felt comfortable with sharing and I wanted to keep his memory to myself, close to my heart.

This loss is just one of the many difficult trials I would face in my life, but it is the one that set the stage for all the others to come. Deep down I knew I would always make it through. It was because of him that my faith grew, and I could find strength in any situation. The Lord was working on paving my path. He was putting together the puzzle pieces of my life to make me whole. This does not mean I did not struggle, but I used counseling and my faith to pull myself out of a period of mourning to acceptance. I have found grace and now know that this was only one chapter in my book of life, one that I would re-visit for courage time and time again. Not one devastating event creates who you are, but it can start to define you and change you in ways you never expected.

A loss such as this will affect many aspects of your life. You gain appreciation for all the little things that may remain meaningless to others. This especially applies to your close friends and family. You pull each of them just a little closer and hold them just a little tighter because you never know what the next days or years has in store for you. This, in turn, makes your relationships stronger. You always remember that difficult situations can always be worse. Most of all your faith grows, no matter what it is and you find yourself surrounded by so many blessings.

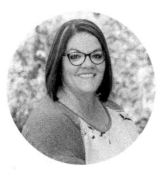

Falon Gervais

Falon Gervais is the loving mother and wife to her two handsome boys and husband Erik. Her son, Owen, is her shining star whom she carries every day in her heart and her rainbow baby, Corbin keeps her on her toes daily.

She has always enjoyed helping others through serving in the National Guard and through her work which has included helping the elderly and children. Falon currently works for a non-profit foster care agency as the program director and is obtaining her master's degree in psychology. She also enjoys volunteering time with Emma's Footprints, helping other loss mothers navigate grief.

Connect with Falon:
https://www.facebook.com/falon.westlake
https://www.instagram.com/falonrai

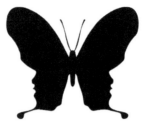

Owen's Story

By Falon Gervais

Owen's story begins long before the pregnancy test was positive. I had always dreamed of being a mother, specifically a mother to a boy. However, I had things I needed to do first: graduate high school, go to college, have fun, live my life, begin a career and be settled in my professional role, fall in love, and live the happily ever after. Now, this was all supposed to happen before I turned thirty but just as the wind blows so did my plan, right out the window on several occasions but one fact remained, I knew I was born to be a mother. The decision to have a baby wasn't a hard one for Erik and I.

Eleven months after going off birth control and one week before turning thirty-two, I took a pregnancy test one Monday morning, not expecting a positive. I was shocked, to say the least, I carried the test to Erik in the kitchen. "So, this happened!" I said. The color drained from his face. He asked me to take another test when I got to work. I did! It was still positive.

We affectionately named the baby nugget, after the first ultrasound. Nugget was due May 5, 2017. I was so overcome by the excitement and anxiety of the upcoming arrival of my baby; it was all-consuming.

Around sixteen weeks, I began to be monitored for an incompetent cervix due to a procedure ten years prior. Every two weeks I got to see my little nugget of joy on that ultrasound screen. When we found out we were having a boy, he needed a name fast. I had several lists of names from years of preparation, but none were made for *this* baby. After several conversations, we decided Owen Lucas would be the perfect name for nugget. We made the transition from nugget to Owen, and by January, everyone called him by his name. This would be music to this mama's ears after his death. He was known, everyone was comfortable with his name and used it, and they still do!

My blood pressure was high, therefore weekly ultrasounds and non-stress tests were started in late February. Seeing and hearing that Owen was thriving eased my mama heart on several occasions. The ultrasound on April 17, 2017, suggested Owen was about 9 lbs. give or take, and at my next doctor's appointment on April 20th my induction was scheduled. I was sweaty and internally checking my to-do list as I left the appointment. It was Thursday, I had three days to finish work and make sure we were ready! I was huge and tired and ready to meet my big boy.

The plan was to arrive at the hospital on Sunday to have Cervadil placed to soften my cervix, be induced Monday morning and a baby by dinnertime. All of which happened, except I had no baby on Monday.

As the early morning hours of Tuesday, April 25th arrived, I was in pain and the epidural wasn't as remarkable as I had been told, nothing about labor was fun or pain-free, but I kept thinking of meeting my baby at the end! Somewhere around 3 am, I decided I was done—if it wasn't time to push, I wanted a C-section. I had lost my ambition, the pain was felt all over, it was time!

I lose parts of the events here. I remember some things so vividly they haunt me and stop me in my tracks when the flashbacks come. Other things I've had to double-check with my husband. I'll probably never recover the memories, and maybe that's okay.

Everything was going smooth. Erik was talking to the doctor, they talked about how much hair Owen had, I joked with Erik about the cottonmouth I was suffering from, and the room was calm apart from my yelling. I pushed for around two hours, but it seemed like twenty minutes when Erik suddenly appeared in front of my face. "You have to focus!" It was like I was zapped into the here and now. Lights came on, codes were called, what seemed like forty people entered my room. I don't recall any conversation, just loud commotion telling me to bare down and push. The lights, the look in everyone's eye—I was determined, in immense pain, and scared shitless.

After what felt like an eternity and several different positions, I felt Owen's lifeless body fall from mine. I have a vision in my head of what this looked like, even though I was facing away from where he was carried. I see it over and over. My heart sank—I was asked to roll over, my work wasn't done. I demanded a minute. I was scared, my baby wasn't crying, I begged and prayed, "Please let my baby cry," and yet, I heard nothing. I asked Erik why my baby wasn't crying, why I couldn't hear him. Erik looked over to Owen and back to me and shook his head. I just knew in my heart he was gone. I was lost. *What do I do now?* I thought. I wanted desperately to be wrong, I wanted to hear his cries but instead, I heard the CPR count. I remember feeling like I was spinning out of control. It was like being stuck on a ride at the fair after everyone left. I felt alone in the room full of people.

The doctor told me I needed to go to the operating room for repair. She looked over to the warmer and said with a shaky voice, "He has a pulse right now, he's alive." As I was being wheeled out of the room, I begged Erik to take pictures and said that I wanted to see him when I was done. He tried his best to convince me that Owen would be okay—I knew otherwise. One of my biggest regrets was turning my head away from Owen as they wheeled me passed him and out of the room. I never saw my son alive. They were prepping to send him to another hospital when his heart stopped again. CPR was performed, questions were asked, and ultimately, Erik agreed that he had been too long without oxygen. Time of death was called at 6:24 am.

I woke in the operating room, my mind high on anesthesia and my gut telling me everything was wrong. I remember the nurse looking me in the eye as I was being wheeled down the hall. I could read the bad news. "Erik has something to tell you," she said. I made eye contact with Erik in the hall, he tried to speak through his tear-stained face. I heard nothing, if he spoke at all, as the tears flowed from my tired eyes. I begged him not to say anything. I knew in my heart Owen was gone, but if someone said it, there was no turning back. I'm not sure if he ever got the words out or I just stopped listening, but vaguely amongst the chaos of nurses, the bright lights, I heard, "He's gone."

Once in my room, I was disoriented but thinking clearly at the same time. I knew what we needed to do, but thoughts swirled around the fact that this was not how this day was supposed to go. The idea that Owen was no longer within me was not something I could make sense of. I knew we needed to call family. I had several messages and missed calls. I messaged my boss and asked her to let everyone know at work, it was easier to tell one person. I couldn't call anyone. I logged into my email and changed my away message from 'maternity leave' to just simply 'leave'. I don't know where this planning came from, it was almost instinctive, which is how I would live for the next few months. If it felt right in the moment I did it. Erik called everyone else. I heard, "Are you sitting down? Falon is fine, but Owen didn't make it," on repeat. I can still hear his calm, quivering voice giving the most devastating news to ever leave his tongue. He didn't look calm from the view on my hospital bed. The sound of my mom screaming through the phone still shakes me.

We had agreed at some point that we wanted more time and wanted to hold Owen, so we asked that no one come until the afternoon if they felt like they had to come. I didn't know what noon meant at that moment; time seemed to have died right along with Owen.

The sweet nurse carried my boy into the room all bundled up, and handed him to me gently. She talked about him as if he was still living, about how cute he was. As she handed his lifeless body to me, I remember feeling this huge sense of pride for birthing a beautiful little boy. I honestly couldn't help but smile. "We did good, Mama," Erik said. This became something we said to each other over and over again in the upcoming weeks. He looked just like a sleeping babe, all bundled up with the pink and blue hospital hat. Looking back at the pictures I see that his color was off, he was bruised on his head and chest, and all the color from his hands and feet was completely drained. I don't remember seeing him like that while I held him. In my mind, he was sleeping. We took pictures that now hang on our walls at home and adorn my desk at work. They are how we introduced Owen's little brother Corbin to him. I'm so thankful for Pat, a complete stranger, who took pictures that morning. She also made molds of his hands and feet, little reminders that he was here and that he lived. I wish I would have held him longer, bathed him, and dressed him in an outfit we brought. I can honestly say I didn't know I needed to ask.

We limited visitors, and we did not have the family meet Owen. At the time, we never even discussed it. I wasn't thinking clearly, I didn't ask, and neither did anyone else. I don't know what is more gut-wrenching — the fact that no one saw him the day he was born or the fact that no one asked. It's easy to get hung up on the 'what if's' now if I take the time to think about it too long. They can consume me if I let them. There is no way to change that now and I'm not about to try. The visitors, they were a blur. I didn't want them there, I would have preferred to hide, or better yet, have them visiting my living baby, the one that was full of life — crying and nursing. Still, a few people came, and some were unexpected. Strangely, I welcomed the unexpected visitors more than those that told us they were coming. They showed their caring hearts without it feeling like they were there because they had to be. It felt good to know that people cared not just about Erik and me, but about Owen as well.

The hospital staff was amazing, my doctors were amazing. The New Life Unit was under construction, but they shut down work for the day, kept me with familiar nurses, and wrapped me in love. I felt their compassion and gentle tones. They shared techniques to ease the pain I would feel in the upcoming days as my milk came in. No one would be able to tell my body that my baby died, and the milk wasn't needed.

We stayed the night at the hospital. I didn't know if I wanted to leave. I was closer to Owen there. Almost safe. There were people outside, people that didn't know what happened.

A nurse walked the halls with me at 3 am. She was so honest and patient, this would be the first time that I heard the term shoulder dystocia. Owen ultimately got his shoulder stuck on my pelvis, leaving him in the birth canal too long, where he was deprived oxygen. She listened and answered my questions. She shared that I had done a good job in the delivery room and the doctor said I was amazing, there was nothing I could have done differently. I didn't know at the time, but I would need these words. I asked for a good therapist. In the blur of what was becoming my life, I was going to need someone to talk to.

As we were being discharged, the nurse asked me if I wanted to take a wheelchair or walk. I chose to walk, on my own two feet with my head held high. Our nurse said, "I knew that's what you would say, you're strong!" I didn't feel strong, I felt nothing. I couldn't hold a thought, yet my mind swirled with words: unanswered questions, broken dreams, sadness, and anger. But still, I was numb.

With a deep breath we were on our way out of the New Life Unit, a walk I had made more times than I could count in the previous weeks, however, this time was different. The walls had lost their color, the elevator that carried my happy soul up on Sunday was delivering my broken heart to my 'after'. We weren't headed home with our brand-new baby boy, we were headed to pick out cemetery plots where we would lay him to rest forever.

The first cemetery was far too expensive and cold, we didn't even leave the car. The funeral director called at just the right time and gave us another place to try.

We drove up through the cemetery, it was beautiful and ready to bloom from all the rain. I was empty but a little butterfly flew over the plot, and I lost it. *This* was his final resting place—it was perfect.

I have spent many hours staring at this little plot of earth. My tears have landed hard while whispers of broken dreams and eternal love floated away with the wind. I have found peace there, and am so thankful we found this spot on our darkest days. If that wasn't already enough for one day, we then headed home to pick out the only outfit our son would ever wear before making the final arrangements at the funeral home. We picked an outfit with the words wild and free on the onesie. I still lose my breath whenever I see similar clothes on other kids. I forgot to take a diaper to the funeral home and felt like a complete failure. Babies wear diapers. Something so little made me feel even more like a failure.

We scheduled the funeral for Saturday so we could close on our new house as planned. Erik wanted to cancel, but I needed something to look forward to. Erik went to close on our house while I had my first few minutes of true alone time since finding out I was pregnant. I wrote a letter to Owen. I needed to put words to paper to make it more tangible. I needed to say I was sorry. Sorry for failing him, sorry that I wasn't able to save him. I know that I could not have done anything differently, but even now, I still catch myself, those feelings of failure are real.

That letter went with him! I wasn't alone long before my best friend showed up again to support me. She took the gel polish off my nails in a kind act of loving support. She showed up and went above and beyond on more than one occasion. For that, I am thankful. She may not have known what to say and she may have been annoying on a few occasions, but she showed up!

We moved into that house just three short weeks after Owen's death, a house that was supposed to be home. Owen's home. We knew what room he was going to sleep in. It was supposed to feel different; it was supposed to be happy, but it took a good nine months and a new baby on the way for me to feel like this was the happy home I envisioned when we toured it.

I stayed on maternity leave for eleven weeks. When I was alone, I looked up other loss stories and mothers like me who managed to survive one, two, five, ten years after the loss of their babies. I needed that hope too. To help, I made a promise to shower every day, it made me feel like I was living while I still felt dead inside.

The concept of time was lost. Days and weeks felt like months. I was afraid to drive, music made me sad, crying made driving difficult, and I would get lost in my head and miss my turn or exit. I struggled to function. While everyone told me I was doing well and better than they expected, they only saw what I would allow them to see. I held strong on the outside, but inside myself and inside my home, I was shattered and barely together.

After returning to work I would crash as soon as I got in my car because I struggled to maintain my professionalism throughout the day. I found it hard to stay focused, I was the queen of multitasking before but when returned my brain felt like mush. Several times my mind would repeat, *Don't they know my baby died, I don't fucking care, there are worse things going on, why are we talking about THIS.* My tolerance for meaningless conversation was limited; my perspective was tainted, and I felt heartless. I wish I could say that went away and those inner dialogues stopped, but they return from time to time.

Through all my confusion, I was able to advocate for myself in ways I would have never imagined my 'before' self to. I went to therapy religiously and return as needed. I went back to the New Life Unit after my six-week appointment to deliver a thank you basket to the staff, because they were affected too. I emailed work before I went back, letting them know my needs and how to support me. I went to a support group where I could say, "I am Owen's mom." Out loud. To a group of people. I showed up to events when I could, and I stayed home when I needed. My heart healed slowly and my new normal took over.

It has been a little over two years. It seems like a lifetime ago. There are days I struggle with who I was and who I am. Still, I think life is unfair, I wanted *my* son here with me, with his dad, with his little brother, I want a complete family picture. I now have to mother Owen in a way that keeps him alive and that works best for my family. We will continue to honor his life and I continue to adjust the way I parent him just as I would if he were growing and thriving. Owen continues to be the reason I jump out of my comfortable space to let the world know he lived.

In losing Owen, I learned that so many people are well-intentioned and want to help, but most of the time they just don't know how. You may need to tell them what you need, even if it is just someone to sit in the darkness, quietly next to you.

You will find joy again; glimmers of hope will seep through your broken cracks. It hurts like hell to miss a piece of you—a lifetime of love spread between Heaven and Earth. Some days will be hard. Grief can slap you off your feet right on to your ass when it's least expected, but there will also be good days—embrace them!

Always remember to give yourself grace. Miss your baby, love your baby, but find a way to love yourself too. You deserve it!

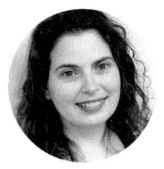

Elizabeth Langer

Dr. Elizabeth Langer is an acupuncturist and chiropractor in Saxonburg, PA, who specializes in helping people with fibromyalgia and chronic pain find relief without medications. She is particularly passionate about helping women with fertility. In her practice, she has found that many women respond favorably to acupuncture and traditional Chinese medicine, which allows them to naturally conceive and have a healthy pregnancy.

Dr. Langer received her Doctor of Chiropractic from New York Chiropractic College in November, 2008 and completed her Master of Science in Acupuncture from the Finger Lakes School of Acupuncture and Oriental Medicine at NYCC in April, 2009.

Connect with Dr. Langer:
https://www.facebook.com/Saxonburg-Acupuncture-Chiropractic-212238068870859/
https://www.linkedin.com/in/elizabeth-langer-52624020/
https://twitter.com/ElizabethLanger

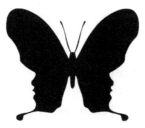

Little Miracles

By Elizabeth Langer

My daughter was the chocolate cake that I never knew I wanted, until I learned I was pregnant. I was starting out in my career and was experiencing a 'whirlwind romance' with my now-husband. We met in Tai Chi (Taiji) class and moved in together after six weeks. About a month after that, we found out that I was pregnant. He was so happy, and the thought of his smile when I told him still makes my heart warm. However, I didn't quite have his confidence. He was like Superman, working and going to school, all while taking care of me. I remember being so scared and so sick that I could barely get out of bed.

At the time, I was working in a very toxic environment and was trapped in a bad contract. I was working six days a week and not making much money. With the constant office drama, and the hostility that was directed at me because I was pregnant, I wanted nothing more than to quit. But I couldn't quit because I would have owed a hefty compensation for the remaining time until my contract was finished. To make matters worse, the morning sickness never stopped. All food nauseated me, and I was rapidly losing weight. Beans became a four-letter word and the smell of vegetables made me gag. The only thing that seemed to sit well was red meat, which was weird because I was a vegan. I got so bad, that thankfully, my boss let me out of my contract and told me I didn't have to pay the compensation fee.

Because I was losing weight and was so sick that I spent most of my time lying in a dark bedroom, some people close to me suggested I terminate the pregnancy because I was "so young" and should "focus on my career." I wanted to say, "Ha! What career!" I felt so betrayed because my husband and I loved this little baby.

Part of the reason I felt so sick was because she decided to start kicking at about two months in and never seemed to stop. I've always been sensitive to energy, so I could never kill this little soul, because we had (and still do) this unspoken and amazing connection. These people advised me to just say that I had "miscarried."

I am happy that I did not listen to that bad advice.

In June 2014, I found out why I was feeling so ill. We had just moved into a new apartment, and as I was rushing to get ready for work, I hit my head on a corner ceiling. I fell to my knees and even though my head spun, I was able to get up and walk to work. When I went to work that day, I discovered that I had forgotten how to write! I also developed a headache that never went away. I went to see a concussion specialist, who ordered an MRI after I performed so poorly on the computerized baseline concussion test that he said, "You're a chiropractor, you should be smarter than this." And sure enough, the MRI found a tumor on my pituitary gland... further testing confirmed that the tumor was due to Cushing's disease. Even though I felt afraid and freaked out that I had this *thing* growing inside my head, I was mostly angry. And I was very angry with my former doctors. After my daughter was born, I began developing the "classic" symptoms of Cushing's disease – I had a hump on my back, hair all over my body (hirsutism), amenorrhea, truncal obesity, and the "moon face." It was exactly like in my medical textbooks… and when I had suggested this to my former PCP, she told me to "lose weight" and "eat less carbs." All the while, the tumor was growing.

My surgery was scheduled for September 15th. I was fortunate because they were able to remove the tumor through my nose. If I would have waited any longer, they would have had to have opened my skull. To me, this was a miracle.

The tumor was embedded into my pituitary gland, so they had to remove a portion of the gland in order to extract it. I was very sick afterwards with hyponatremia—a condition where your sodium levels are dangerously low. Looking back, I believe what made everything easier was the big miracle that happened while I was still in the hospital.

No visitors were allowed in the recovery unit at night. I was alone and in a lot of pain. So much so that I was afraid that I would die. Even though I was in the special ward with a wonderful doctor, this was the same hospital that my cousin died due to negligence. On top of the fear, I was so angry. When I thought about it, I had been angry for a very long time… Not just because of the tumor, but anger had always served as a baseline emotion and I didn't want to die with this anger in my heart. So, I prayed. If you ever watched Joel Osteen, I prayed that little prayer that he always says at the end, and I asked God to come into my heart.

Lord Jesus, come into my heart, wash me clean… I make you my Lord and Savior.

And God came to me. I felt him in the room and saw him clearly in my mind. You could say it was the Percocet, but I don't think so. He assured me that everything would be okay, that he was always with me, and that he would give me my face back. This experience transformed me from the inside out and continues to shape my path.

I wasn't worried three months later when I didn't menstruate, because I figured that my body had been through such a shock. But at thirty-two years old, my endocrinologist broke the news that I was going through menopause. She said that it was time to harvest my eggs. It didn't hit me at first, and I told her that I would really have to think about it. Chiropractic and acupuncture are both physical jobs, so I was uncertain of my professional future. And faced with medical debts on top of student loans, I didn't see how we could afford another baby at that point, my body was so weak; I didn't see how I could possibly carry a healthy baby to term. One night I couldn't breathe, so we went to the hospital where I had a breathing treatment, and then went to work the next day, with the hospital bracelet tucked under my sleeve. I needed this job and I had to work. My husband had just lost his job because he had been trying to take care of everything - our daughter, our home, and me, and had taken too much time off. I knew it wasn't the right time to have a baby, but it didn't stop me from wanting one.

I went home and held my daughter, and was (and still am) grateful for this miracle. But I still cried bitter tears at my body's 'failure'. Even though it was a miracle that I was even able to conceive, my heart still hurt. My husband and I were both only children, so that's probably why we both wanted a big family. I thought about the medications that were necessary to keep me alive. And I was worried about the toxicity that could carry over. For financial reasons, we decided to wait until I was stronger.

I began to delve into the interrelationship between health and fertility. Infertility is considered to be a symptom of an underlying problem in traditional Chinese medicine (TCM). Whether the patient has a pre-existing condition, such as endometriosis, an unhealthy lifestyle, or is missing a portion of their pituitary gland, the result is failure to conceive. Acupuncture is merely a tool of TCM to be used to increase health and establish balance. In order to have a healthy baby, a woman must first have a healthy body. Since Qi is the vital substance responsible for life, having an abundance of Qi in the right areas of the body is essential for conception.

When I work with women to help them conceive, I usually work with them at each stage of their cycle. However, I didn't have a cycle, so I was unsure of what to do. In addition to acupressure and acupuncture, I began to change my diet to better boost my Qi. I listened to what my body needed, and experimented with taking different supplements, such as vitamin D3, a B complex, and chelated magnesium. I adopted a gentle exercise regimen of Taiji and yoga, trying to nourish myself, while not overexerting. And even though I wasn't able to menstruate, I felt as though I was growing stronger every day.

Two years later, when I felt strong enough, I asked my OBGYN, who is also an acupuncturist, about having a baby. My husband had been working steadily and I was starting to find stability in my practice. We even found a wonderful sitter for our daughter!

She smiled warmly and told me that my uterus and ovaries were "perfectly healthy." They just weren't communicating with the remaining portion of my pituitary gland. She gave me the name of a doctor who specialized in high-risk pregnancies. High-risk… meaning I would have to replace my current medications with *another* set of medications, in addition to tons of bed rest. Since my body no longer made cortisol, along with the other hormones necessary for a healthy pregnancy, carrying a baby could have a negative impact on my heart and kidneys. There were so many unknown factors that threatened to jeopardize not just my health, but my very life. Would the combination of carrying a baby and the cocktail of drugs and hormones send me backwards in my progress? If so, then how could I parent my daughter? And what effect could these new drugs and hormones have on a developing baby?

As much as I wanted another baby, I realized that I wasn't ready to chance losing everything that I currently had, such as the close relationship with my little girl. I realized how blessed I truly was and began to release the pain. Of course I was sad, and yes, a little bit angry. But I didn't need another baby to complete our family and I didn't need another baby to complete myself. The waves of gratitude for my magical little gift and the fact of my transformation overtook the feelings of self-pity and despair.

Once I was able to release the feelings of anger and sadness, I was able to focus on my daughter while getting stronger physically and emotionally. I always enjoyed working with fertility, but after making peace with my own journey, I was better able to help others. And I think that through helping others, I am better able to heal myself.

Something that I have always believed, but never realized the power of was this – a family doesn't necessarily have to be who you are biologically related to. There are a lot of kids in this world who need loving homes. Moving forward, when the time is right, we would love to open our hearts and our homes to kids who need them. And if it is in God's will that I should get pregnant, then I will have to leave that up to him.

Sometimes acceptance is the first step in healing. And when you feel grateful for what you have, instead of pining for what you don't, your heart fills with a warmth that can replace the pain if you allow it. And that's when miracles can happen!

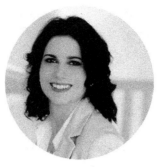

Cathy McKinnon

Cathy McKinnon is the founder of Wellness Warrior Coaching, offering a combination of wellness and life coaching services. She works with ambitious women to create personalized success rituals to gain more energy, strength, beauty and confidence along their journey to optimal living. Cathy came to this career through her own transformation and battles with weight loss, cancer, divorce and infertility. Now she shares her learnings to help other women avoid the same pitfalls she did and start to show up unapologetically as their authentic selves. Cathy has been featured on several podcasts including Fearless Woman (episode 56), Success through Failing (episode 152), and A Sacred Space with Katie.

Connect with Cathy:
www.facebook.com/wellnesswarriorcoaching
www.instagram.com/wellnesswarriorcoaching
www.pinterest.com/wwarriorcathy

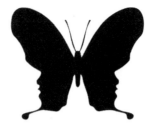

Intuitive Guidance

By Cathy McKinnon

We grow up thinking motherhood is a natural part of life. It's a key component of being a woman, or so I thought growing up.

I remember the first time I found out I was pregnant. I honestly didn't believe it and took test after test to confirm. I had been on birth control for about ten years at that point, so I really had no idea what 'normal' was. I didn't have morning sickness. I just felt 'off'. This was the beginning of me learning to trust my intuition.

It took a few weeks for reality to sink in, then things started to spiral out of control.

After my initial doctor appointment, I went for my first ultrasound. At approximately eight weeks I found out there was no heartbeat and that I had miscarried. The doctor suggested (and at this point I was unaware of other options) that I let the miscarriage happen naturally. Let's just say for me, for my body, that was a *horrible* idea. I remember stumbling down the stairs at 1 a.m. to stand in a steaming shower, trying not to pass out from the pain and blood loss. No one knew I was pregnant, so who could I call at 1 a.m. to tell them I thought I was dying. A week had passed, and I grew weaker by the day. The doctor ordered a surgical dilation and curettage, commonly referred to as a D&C.

I didn't know how to process the emotions that came with that first miscarriage. I was shocked to have been pregnant in the first place. So, was it shocking to have lost the pregnancy? It was a loss of life. A swirling of questions and emotions that I kept to myself as I didn't think anyone else would understand.

After that, I had decided that I really wanted a baby and I was done putting it on the back burner for my career.

The next pregnancy came as a pleasant surprise. I thought this was it, I was better prepared this time, so it would work out. Right? Well, I was wrong. At the ten-week mark, there was no heartbeat. This time I couldn't just wait for things to happen naturally and I scheduled the D&C.

With a heavy heart, I became depressed and questioned myself. What was I doing wrong? Was there something someone didn't tell me? I felt that no one understood and therefore I had no one to turn to talk through the swirling thoughts in my head. My partner was stoic about it and therefore did not offer up a comforting shoulder. As we often do these days, I started to Google. What was I missing about this critical component of womanhood?

After the third miscarriage and the third D&C, I was becoming a shell of myself. Going through the motions, exhausted physically and mentally. I was depressed and angry. *Why me? What did I do? What was I doing wrong?*

I was in such a bad emotional state that seeing babies in stores or in commercials would cause me to breakdown. Attending baby showers for close friends was not something I could face, and I felt like an awful friend. I wanted to be happy for my friends but could not face the events.

Doctors told me I was young, I had time, it was not unheard of, but I didn't feel consoled. I didn't feel right... again I had that sinking feeling that something was off. I didn't know what 'it' was but I just felt *something* was wrong.

After three miscarriages, the doctors started to take me seriously and I started to have additional testing and work ups done. It was at an annual appointment with my OBGYN that she noticed a nodule on my thyroid, she played this off, saying we are in the nodule belt of the U.S., that it's not uncommon. However, she still wanted me to go to an endocrinologist. I remember thinking to myself, *not another doctor! Who has time to keep taking off work for all these appointments? Besides you just told me it's nothing...*

I went to the endocrinologist, who also thought that it was nothing, but he ordered a biopsy just in case, which was one of the most painful experiences of my life. Five biopsies were taken from my neck that day from a nodule that was less than two centimeters in size. The level of anxiety I experienced drove me crazy. All I wanted was the all-clear so I could check the box and continue the path to have my baby. The infertility specialist was awaiting this report before he would proceed with my treatments.

The biopsy was done on a Friday and I called to get the results the following Wednesday. "Nothing yet," said the nurse. Friday was the start of a long, Labor Day weekend. I had my Harley and was ready to spend the weekend at the Harley Anniversary party in Milwaukee. I was eager to celebrate a clean report.

A few hours before I was to leave work for the big celebration, I had not yet heard from the doctor. I called and was told by the nurse that they would call me back. The nurse called me back and asked if I could come in to see the doctor on the Tuesday following the holiday weekend. At that point, I knew something was terribly wrong. If it was negative they would be able to give me the all-clear over the phone.

I demanded the doctor call me back as at that point it was evident that something was terribly wrong! I had a sick feeling in my stomach. The doctor came to the phone and stated that it was not his preferred method to discuss things like this over the phone. I begged him to tell me. I *needed* to know.

Then, he finally spat it out. The biopsy was positive for papillary cancer. I hung up the phone and just sat there, dumbfounded. Two doctors had essentially convinced me that it was benign, it was nothing. I spent that weekend in an absolute haze. I didn't tell anyone except my partner as I did not know how to process the result myself.

I met with the surgeon right after the holiday weekend. I sat in her office, staring blankly as she told me the plan of action. I had to get a copy of the biopsy report in my hands, I had to see it to believe it. Somehow seeing the words myself would make a difference, or that's what I told myself.

At no time during all of this did anyone ask how I was doing mentally or emotionally. I felt like a number, going through the motions of doctor visits, surgical procedures, and lab tests. My partner saw me going through the motions but again did not offer emotional support.

The next morning, I woke with a sense of calm, a path of action was defined, and it was time to get this over with so that I could have my baby. I had surgery to have my entire thyroid removed, which meant a lifetime of prescription medication.

The surgery was much more painful than I had thought it would be, and the pain was compounded by the layoff notification I received from my employer between my diagnosis and surgery.

I recovered from the surgery in an empty house, not knowing the future or my ability to have my baby. I spent my days trying to recover from the surgery, going to follow up appointments, and Googling my prognosis (do not do this). It was a massive rollercoaster of emotions and yet no medical provider I saw asked,

"How are you?" If no one was talking about it, then it just must be me and my coping skills, right? That's certainly how it felt.

A year after my radiation treatment, I was cleared to again begin to try to conceive. I was working with an infertility specialist at this point, dealing with lab tests, medications, injections and a routine that seemed overwhelming.

It will all be worth it, I kept telling myself as I tried to manage the schedule; disregarding my declining mental health.

Off the bat, I was able to conceive; however, the pattern followed suit and I was not able to maintain the pregnancy... another miscarriage and D&C.

Yet another miscarriage and D&C followed in the subsequent months. My doctor advised me to take a break, give my body a breather. In my head, I was thinking about menopause looming and my cancer treatments affecting my ability to conceive. I wasn't getting younger. I had to keep going. I had to get myself as healthy as possible—mind, body, and energy.

I did a lot of research. I talked to mothers, doctors, and experts. I wanted to do anything I could to make my pregnancy a success. I took the vitamins, drank the tea, tracked the calendar, ate specific foods. I became obsessed.

I started my next round of injections and held my breath that this time would somehow be different.

Since I have no thyroid, I had to have constant testing of my thyroid levels. One round of tests showed that my levels were through the roof. The doctor immediately wanted to stop the round of fertility drugs and ordered me to see the endocrinologist.

I questioned what all this could mean. The doctor didn't want to say for sure, but there was a possibility that my cancer was back. I felt so much anger, so much rage; I was following all the instructions, I was doing *everything* right, and now after giving myself countless injections, my cancer might be back?!

I went back to the cancer center, where the doctor ordered labs and a radioactive iodine scan. I heard nothing from the lab results so I figured everything must be okay and I continued through the motions of the scan. As with anytime you ingest radiation, I did not feel well for days afterward. I thought this was the effect of the radiation and the decrease of the fertility medications mixing to create an awful feeling. By the end of the week, I still felt like death. I called the doctor's office to see if this was normal.

I asked her if the lab work indicated anything. Suddenly, the phone went silent. I remember asking her repeatedly, "What did the pregnancy test say? Her only response was, "The doctor will call you back." Then I knew... I had radiation treatment while pregnant. The best the doctor could offer at this point was, "I'm sorry." There was no way to know how this would impact my unborn child.

When I found out I was pregnant, I was hesitant, afraid to be happy. *What if this time will be no different?* I said to myself.

The night before my ultrasound I was nervous, this often was the point where I found out that I had miscarried. I tossed and turned that night, but when I did sleep, I had the most vivid dream where I learned I was carrying twins.

With my family history, this was a strong possibility. My mother is a twin and my partner's mother is a twin.

As I headed to my appointment that morning, I was filled with anxiety. What would 1 see? Would the typical news be delivered that I was losing the baby? Was my dream telling me something that there was a bigger message here? So many questions in my mind as I drove to the doctor's office.

There they were on the ultrasound, two heartbeats! I was happy and overwhelmed—double the joy. I was not yet ready to tell anyone, I was silenced with fear. It didn't help that my partner didn't support or comfort me at all. In fact, he barely said a word. This left me with even more anxiety knowing the person I needed the most was completely unavailable. Why was I the only one riddled with all of this anxiety and fear?

Due to the radiation exposure, I was sent to a neonatal specialist in downtown Chicago and went through testing. The end result was that they didn't think there would be any danger to the babies, however, there was truly no way to tell. How can you quell anxiety when left with an open-ended statement regarding the health of the babies you are carrying?

I wanted to keep this secret until we passed the twelve-week safe zone, which coincided with my mother's birthday.

A few weeks before the big reveal I had planned, I was going up the stairs in the hallway at work and suddenly doubled over in pain. All I thought was, *Shit this is it, it's all over.* I called the doctor, who asked me to come in immediately.

The news was mixed. One of the twins did not make it, but the other still had a strong heartbeat.

For the remainder of the pregnancy, I remained anxious about the health of the baby I was carrying. Would I lose him too? Would he be impacted by the radiation? Would he have physical or mental challenges from the radiation? It was not a healthy amount of stress/anxiety for a pregnant woman.

June 21st 2011, I walked laps trying to get my baby boy excited to make his entrance into the world. I walked through the anxiety, fear and joy. He would be finally be here!! Followed by oh my god he is going to be here!

5 years of waiting, crying, and pushing my body to its limits. More appointments and procedures than I could count to get me to this day.

On June 22nd, 2011, I was induced and my miracle baby boy arrived into this world. I got to hold him and grieve for his lost twin. All the emotions one could feel were felt in those first 24 hours.

I am grateful for my baby boy every day, how he saved me, how he brought me to this place in my journey, how he teaches me to savor the moments in the present.

This journey taught me so much about myself, but one thing stands out: do not neglect your holistic health. Do not rely on doctors if you feel something is off, ask the questions, get a second opinion, and push for answers. Ensure you are comfortable with your doctor. Your energies must jive. If you are uncomfortable, find another provider! Find a tribe of health care providers, friends, and family that can support all aspects of your journey-mental and physical. You cannot be your optimal self by ignoring your mental health. If your doctor is not taking the time to discuss it; find a supportive ear and work through all those emotions, thoughts and anxieties. You have to advocate for your best life!

I swore when I was blessed with my son that I would do what I had to do to show up as best I could for him, he deserved it. He is my miracle baby.

As I write this chapter, I am so proud of moments where he shows the kindness in his soul, saying things to me unprompted like, "Mom, meetings can be replaced ; I can't be replaced …I'm so glad you step out of meetings when I want to talk to you."

It was all worth it.

I see you. I hear you. I am you.

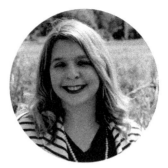

Kara Peters

Kara Peters is a debut author, who has an ambition to soar as a writer. She enjoys reading and writing inspirational and motivational material. It is truly her passion to engage in uplifting projects for others, while always remaining authentic and humble.

She is a wife to an amazing husband Joshua, and together they have five beautiful children. She holds a Bachelor's Degree in Interdisciplinary Studies and wishes to pursue a career as a writer in addition to going back to school to study Journalism. She hopes to always encourage her readers.

Connect with Kara:
www.facebook.com/KaraPeters
https://www.instagram.com/KaraPeters

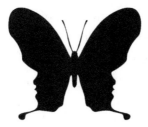

The Essence of My Sunflower

By Kara Peters

Miscarriage. That one word changed my life forever. Hearing this word from the doctor that my baby growing inside of me was no longer here was devastating—a complete shock. Through my sadness, I had peace that my precious baby was in the loving arms of Jesus. However, my heart will always be broken that my husband and I will never get to meet my child and my other children will never get to play with their sibling. The guilt still consumes me today that if I just did something different maybe my child would be here today. As a mother, I will go to the ends of the earth to protect my children and provide the best life for them. Although I will never understand why, I know in my heart that God had a plan and reason for allowing this to happen. My unwavering faith and family helped me get through this incredibly hard time. I pray that through my experience, I can help others find comfort in the time of loss and hope as time goes on.

Life was so busy and great! My husband and I were blessed with three beautiful children. They were, and still are, the entire reason we work as hard as we do and make the hard choices necessary for their future. Our oldest, Elizabeth was about to wrap her school year as an ambitious first grader. We were in the month of early April, so she had less than two months left until the exciting arrival of summer vacation. Having two young boys was amazing, and a challenge to say the least. I dedicated my time to being a stay at home mother, as this was what was best suited for our family at the time. During all of this wonderful craziness, we were given an unexpected surprise, our fourth baby was coming. This was confirmed by the bold plus sign on the pregnancy test. Although we felt a little overwhelmed, my husband and I both were overjoyed with the news of welcoming a new life into our loving family.

I was only a few weeks along when we discovered this blessing and we shared the news with all of our loved ones. It was perfect timing as spring was approaching and I was starting off the season of newness and growth all around us with the uplifting feeling of a new little human growing inside of me. For anyone out there who has expected a little bundle of joy, you know the inundation of emotions that permeate through you. For those who have yet to experience this euphoric feeling, the best way I can describe it is a combination of joy, tears, and nervousness. In this stage, I could not help but to get ahead of myself with my thoughts and ponder what the gender was and how we were going to decorate the nursery. Everything that involves bringing a new baby into our lives was at the forefront of my thoughts.

About three weeks later, everything changed. The excitement we were embracing was suddenly put to a halt when an incident occurred. My sister-in-law, Nicole and I were walking with our children at a local park. Between her children and mine, it was more of a relaxed slow walk, so nothing intense was happening. It was a beautiful sun-filled day and the water was completely breathtaking to look at as we walked further down the trails. As we were walking back, I started to feel off. I brushed the feeling aside assuming fatigue was just setting in a little. When we returned to the parking lot a restroom stop was completely necessary for our children and myself. Having been pregnant three times before, I was very familiar with the urgency of a full bladder. I am sure all you other mothers who have experienced any length of pregnancy can vouch for that. The bathroom trip was going as smoothly as possible with as many children as we had between the two of us, until I noticed blood. My heart stopped and emotions started getting the best of me, so I immediately tried to calm myself down, as I did not want to worry the children. I reasoned with my own mind that it was normal and a little bleeding can happen at times. At least that is what I was praying for. In all three of my other pregnancies nothing like that had ever occurred.

The following week was Mother's Day. We spent the day with our children and my family at the local zoo. Ideally, this was a fantastic idea as we were all excited to have some real quality family time with one another. The heat was unbearable that day. I can't even put into words the physical and emotional turmoil that transpired on that specific day. What I had prayed was a possible normal pregnancy experience, turned into an absolute unacceptance of what was about to occur. As the journey through the zoo continued, I felt painful cramps start to infiltrate my entire midsection. That indescribable sinking feeling that the absolute worst scenario that could possibly happen was happening, and there was nothing I could say or do to stop it. My baby was dead! I knew it, and that shook me at my very core.

I remembered back to my ultrasound after the spotting incident. At that time my baby was still alive, however, they were concerned with the size. My mother was with me that day and I do not know how I would have taken the news without her unwavering support. It was back to the present moment as I slowly brought myself back into reality. The extensive pain was increasing by the moment and I grabbed my husband's arm. The last thing I wanted to do was ruin the day and what we were attempting to create beautiful family memories. However, I knew there was no going back and no controlling the inevitable. If I could insert a tearful emoji here I really would as my hands are literally shaking and tears are filling my eyes as I think back and relive the loss. This particular trip we were accompanied by my parents Jim and Shirley, my younger sister Krista, brother-in-law Chris, and my younger brother Jimmy. My family was made aware of the level of pain that was encompassing my entire body as they rushed over to help. They all agreed it was time to get me to the car. In my head I was terrified and screaming! *Why?! On Mother's Day, just to add to the wound!* I am the mother, the one person that my baby could depend on, and it was dying inside of me. The overwhelming guilt seeped through me, and to be honest still surfaces to this very day. That horrific feeling that was reality, I could not protect my own baby! My husband, Joshua and I left the zoo and took our other children to drop off at my parent's house so we could go to the hospital from there. However, by the time we entered their house my pain level was much more than I could bear. I crawled onto my parent's bed (as it was the closest comfortable spot), and my miscarriage proceeded.

A while later, I was numb from emotional distress and physical pain. We went to the hospital and they confirmed what I already knew was the fate of my unborn child. He or she was gone. The doctor who broke the news to me was not very compassionate and just said, "The fetus is gone." I looked him square in the face, with all sorts of emotions combined together and responded by saying, "You mean my baby is dead?" He then ignored that statement and said with an annoyingly cheerful voice, "Well, you can always try again!" I wanted to scream, punch a wall, anything. Yes, realistically we could eventually try to conceive again if we so chose, however, this baby cannot be replaced! I couldn't believe the lack of compassion and wanted the doctor to exit the room immediately.

Through it all, the one thing that kept me from breaking down beyond repair was my husband by my side. He unequivocally loved me and nurtured me every step throughout the whole process. I know it is cliché, but he will always be my solid rock. The one that God has put with me to stand by my side through everything life will present to us. Looking back, I really struggle with how difficult this whole ordeal was for him. Having had three children before this, I know all too well his overwhelming excitement every time he learned were about to bring another life into the world. To this day he gets choked up when we discuss the heartbreak we carry as a result of that day. I think it is crucial that we remember the father's during these times, as they have suffered a loss as well. In addition, they have to watch the one they love suffering through immeasurable pain. Check on them, pray for them, usually they mask their feelings in an attempt to be strong for the mother. However, they should not be overlooked. Both my husband and I began the healing process together, with God at the center of it all.

The night of my loss, after arriving home and resting for a while, I started the phone calls to inform friends and family of the tragic occurrence that had just taken place. I was truly not expecting, or wanting anything, other than to convey the message that I will be in mourning for the time being. I knew this was going to forever affect me, and I just needed to hear comforting voices. My sister Krista, and her husband Christopher, along with my little brother and my parents were as you remember already with me consoling me that day as everything was taking place. So, I called others in my circle I am closest too. Two people I really needed to hear from were my sisters-in-law, Nicole and Michelle. They both mean the world to me as well and are always there through every aspect of life. They were both filled with heartwarming compassion. Michelle had previously lost a baby of her own and could very much relate to my situation. I also called my Aunt Shelly, whom I could not literally live life without, and my best friends, Musiette, Jocelyn, and Leah. All of the conversations were filled with heartfelt condolences and were so immense and genuine. They all make me so grateful to have an amazing support system, something I pray all of you reading this have in your lives as well. I received an act of kindness that evening as Musiette and Nicole came over to just be present in my emotional state. They were trying to lift my spirits, which was not going to happen that evening but was an amazing gesture and I will forever appreciate the effort. My sister in law, Nicole even brought me ice cream and a beautiful sunflower, the flower that would become my décor piece in memory of my baby. The countless acts of kindness and encouragement touched my very soul. No amount of saying thank you will ever be enough to emphasize the peace they brought to me on that dark day.

I truly and wholeheartedly can say I was humbled by this experience, as I was that person who thought a pregnancy loss could never happen to me. After all, I was blessed to have carried three healthy babies to term before. Elizabeth, Noah, and Jacob… all three of my children were held much closer that evening and I vowed then and there to never take for granted the joy they bring to my life.

Three months after my miscarriage I actually learned that I was pregnant again! This was not planned and came as a complete shock. My husband and I were overjoyed, however, we felt a nervousness never felt before. We prayed together for a strong and healthy pregnancy, and that the baby would not only survive, but thrive. Since the loss was still heavy on our hearts, we decided to hold off on announcing the pregnancy until I hit the three-month mark. Nine months later, I delivered a beautiful healthy baby boy, our little Luke. That was not the end of our news! Three and a half months after that I found out I was expecting again! We were so scared, five children! However, we could not contain our nerves and waited again to reveal our newest blessing. We knew this one would complete our family and I gave birth to a healthy and strong, gorgeous baby girl! We named her Alana, at the request of our oldest daughter, Elizabeth. We allowed her to pick the name because she had a rough time with the miscarriage and trying to comprehend everything. She was convinced our little baby in heaven was a girl so we named the baby Gabrielle. And just in case it was a boy, we chose the name Gabriele as well.

My faith was tested the day I lost my baby, but I have since overcome any doubt. In the present day, I still have guilt issues, as previously talked about. I question myself that if I wouldn't have pushed myself so hard on the walks that my baby would have survived. No matter what people say to try to bring me out of the guilt, I do not know if it is feasible to think that it will ever leave me. However, I truly encourage every woman and her significant other who experiences a loss, to complete what I call a healing project. For me, it was an idea sparked by my sister in completing a shadow box with the only ultrasound picture I ever received of my baby. It was utterly significant to reaching a certain closure I had not felt before. She was with me through every part of this project and we included my daughter Elizabeth as well! The project sits in my dining room on a shelf with a beloved angel statue given to me by my father-in-law, Mike, and my mother-in-law, Cheryl. And surrounding those items are sunflowers. This was a spark of happiness and color, in a dim situation.

For those of you who endure a loss of a precious baby, please reach out to those who emotionally support you. Maybe even engage in a healing project of your own from your heart. It is something that you will always remember as a tribute to your son or daughter. God bless every single one of you, and your precious babies, gone too soon. You are loved and valued! My greatest heartfelt thank you to everyone in my corner, and I pray all of you reading this have a loving support system as well, no matter how big or small. You are also always welcome to connect with me through my contact information.

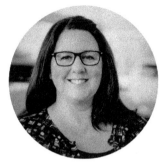

Jennifer Philip

Jennifer Philip is a self-proclaimed work in progress.

A passionate mother and wife, she loves to travel and is always looking for that next adventure. Having traveled around the world working on cruise ships, she believes that traveling not only educates but enlightens the soul.

Jennifer has journaled for most her life, but in these last few years has begun to share her thoughts through her blog, *The Female Project*. Through writing and putting herself 'out there', her followers have found her to be straight forward and brutally honest. She shares the hard, untold stories that many are afraid to reveal, with the hopes that others don't feel as alone and can avoid the pain she has endured.

The Female Project has allowed her to connect with thousands of women all over the world. She is currently exploring alcohol abuse in women and writes on other topics such as infertility, depression, anxiety, marriage, and motherhood.

Her community of followers help reinforce her belief that women raising up women is the most powerful movement there is, and when we share and learn from each other we can change the world.

Connect with Jennifer:
https://www.facebook.com/jennifer.philip.9
https://thefemaleproject.com/
https://www.facebook.com/thefemaleprojectdotcom/

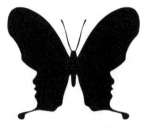

The Miracle of Unanswered Prayers

By Jennifer Philip

I have wanted to be a mom as far back as I can remember. Getting married and having a big fancy wedding were never part of my daydreams. But I would dream about the day I would become a mother. I would dream about what my child would look like. What we would talk about. How we would cuddle together and how much I would love him or her.

I lost my virginity at a young age as I was in a very long term, committed relationship and I remember hating taking the pill. I was always sick and just never felt good. I stopped taking it and being stupid, rarely used any other type of protection. Being intimate was always me taking a 'chance' and hoping for the best.

I never got pregnant.

As a teenager, I played all the scenarios in my mind of what would happen if I did become pregnant. What would I do? Who would I tell? Would I be able to keep it?

I wish I could go back to that young girl and tell her to stop worrying. *You won't get pregnant.*

The months turned into years and as I entered into my twenties having never practiced safe sex, I remember having mixed emotions. On the one hand, I felt like one lucky girl for always taking the chance and never getting pregnant, but in the back of my mind, I felt disappointment and wonder as to why I never did get pregnant. In my rational mind, I knew that the fact that I hadn't gotten pregnant was a good thing, but as woman it nagged at me and I remember feeling worried. Worried and nervous as to why my body didn't do what a woman's body should.

Years passed and my desire to become a mother got stronger. So strong that I walked away from my fiancé three weeks before we were to get married. At this time in my life, I was working on cruise ships and traveling the world. I was in a whirl-wind relationship with an officer on a ship and after two years together we flew to England to gather his family and friends and then head to Canada to get married.

I remember his mood changing on the way to England. He was distant and I felt a sinking feeling in my gut. When we were finally home, I asked him what was going on. I was worried and confused. He proceeded to tell me that he didn't want to have children. That his life was the sea and he wanted to marry me and have me share that life with him, but children were not part of his dream. Wow… this came out of left field and I remember sitting there feeling like I could not believe this was happening. My mind was spinning. Why he waited to tell me this at this moment still baffles me. But he continued to say that although a life of travel and adventure would make me happy, ultimately, I would be missing the one thing I want, and that was to be a mother and he couldn't lie to me anymore. He didn't want kids, end of story. I sat across from him and my mind was racing. We were supposed to get married in three weeks. People were coming from all over. Everything was paid for. Honeymoon booked. But when I looked across the table all my feelings changed. I couldn't get married to someone with the hopes of changing their minds. My body was cold and empty, but we ended it very simply. No kids, no marriage.

There was literally no conversation or negotiations.

It was done. I moved on.

In some ways, that relationship was a blessing because it cemented how important motherhood was to me.

The irony in all of this was that years later I would fall deeply in love with the man who stood by me through all of this, and would have to have the same conversation with him, but in reverse. I would be asking him to make a decision. I had to tell the most important person in my life that I may be broken. That I may not be able to conceive.

I remember how upset he used to get with me when we were dating. I would get my period and cry. He didn't understand that as the years went on, I began to really start questioning why I wasn't getting pregnant.

When he proposed and we were planning on getting married, it was a conversation that I felt I needed to bring up. Would he be okay if we never had children? We both wanted four, but what if it wasn't meant to be? He had dreams of a big family and assured me that his love for me was strong enough to go through this challenge together and we would tackle the good and the bad head-on.

As soon, as we were married, we put all our energy into trying to conceive. We were not just having sex or making love, we were focused on getting pregnant. We started to have sex three times a day. And let me tell you, it is definitely not like the movies. It wasn't romantic by any means. Instead, it felt like a stressful chore.

The hardest part was that every month I was still getting a period. Right on time, each and every month. And each month was the same emotional rollercoaster. I would often curl up in a ball on my bed and just lay there crying. But then it was time to stand up and wipe the tears away and start again. Each new month starting off hopeful and positive. With new plans in place of healthy living and doing all the tricks out there to get pregnant. We tried having sex with my feet in the air, then with a pillow under my butt, wearing socks was supposed to help or taking cough syrup. None of them worked, but we tried them all, always hopeful.

Any woman who is trying to get pregnant knows that feeling of disappointment when they are trying to conceive. But when months and years go by the mental mind game that goes on can make you feel like you are going crazy. I was constantly looking at the calendar and counting. Always thinking, this time it's going to happen. I could convince myself each month that I was pregnant. My breasts were sore, or I felt nauseous or I was tired… and then blood. Tears. Try again.

Eventually, I decided I wanted to see a fertility specialist and my husband was on board with it.

When you go to see the doctor there are so many forms to fill out. They needed to know everything about us physically. Blood was taken, urine examined, and sperm scrutinized. Once this was done we got to see the doctor. There he reviewed everything with us and let us know that there was nothing wrong with us. This was horrible news. I wanted there to be something. For there to be an explanation, but instead, all he could tell us was that we were two healthy individuals who should be able to have children. I knew that we couldn't just take this answer and walk out the door. I told him… I didn't ask… I *told* him, regardless of the results, I was willing to pay and move forward with fertility treatment. I spoke in a very confident, sure manner. Letting him know that I wasn't leaving until a plan was in place. He looked at the chart and then looked at my husband and me and said he understood and would proceed with us because I was thirty-three and mature enough to start the process.

After that initial visit, I never saw him again. I ended up becoming the closest with the nurse I would see every day. Her dedication and commitment to her patients blew me away. She worked every day, 365 days a year!

Everything about fertility treatment is unromantic and anti-sexual. When you get a third party involved it took some of the pressure off at the beginning. I was hopeful and glad that there were experts who could monitor me and be with us through the journey. And with someone helping us, we went back to normal lovemaking with the hopes that with both science and sex something would eventually work.

When we started I had to be at the clinic by 7 am every day to have an internal ultrasound to see the size of my eggs. They were monitored and watched as they grew. I remember being excited during our first session. Even though we lived in the country, an hour away from the clinic, I still woke up each morning ready to make the drive in the cold, dark winter mornings. When I would arrive, I would have my blood and urine taken. Then I would get changed and wait anxiously in the ultrasound room for the nurse. I remember the room being very comforting. The lights were off and the glow from the ultrasound machine made the room feel like a safe place. Then the nurse would come in an insert an apparatus inside me and we would look at my eggs together. She was always positive and encouraging and excited about how healthy my eggs looked. It's amazing how excited you can get looking at their own eggs.

That morning routine went on for about two weeks before the nurse sent me home with a needle to inject into my belly at a specific time the next day. Giving myself a needle in the stomach freaked me out. I remember not being able to do it and having to lie on the bed and ask my husband to inject me. It didn't hurt nearly as much as I had made it out in my mind. Then we had to wait for another twenty-four hours before we headed into the clinic... together.

Besides our initial interview with the doctor, this was my husband's first time joining me on this journey. He didn't have to go every morning like I did and he hadn't built a relationship with the nurse like I had. He was mostly curious and eager to do his part. When we arrived at the clinic at 7 am, we were the only ones there. It was silent and very clinical. I remember he was given a cup to fill with sperm and was put into an examination room.

I really felt for my husband at this point because there was a lot of pressure on him to 'perform' and to get a good quantity of sperm to fill the cup. The examination room he was in was a pregnancy exam room with pictures of pregnant women and babies breastfeeding on the walls. Nothing to help someone get 'in the mood' to do the deed if you know what I mean. I think he thought the room would be set up for a man to do what he needs to do. Like in the movies where they have videos and magazines. That was not the case. Instead, I could hear him trying to make something happen, but was struggling. I knocked on the door to see how it was going... he said it was going nowhere.

When the nurse came to check on us, she let us know that I could go into the room with him to 'help'. Now I felt like the pressure was on me. I remember thinking about how are we going to make this happen. Someone was outside the door, we were nervous and simply uncomfortable. I then had a 'now or never moment' and took off my clothes and tried to get intimate in the most ridiculous situation. I pulled out my bag of tricks and bang he was ready to go. We ended up having sex on the examination table with full concentration on pulling out just in time for us to gather all the semen in the cup. Success!

Now that the pressure was off my husband, he got fully involved with the rest of the procedure. The nurse took the specimen, examined it under a microscope and lets us know that my husband had great sperm. There were millions of them, and they were all very active, moving fast and in the right direction. Hearing this made him proud, and I kind of giggled inside. So now we had great sperm and great eggs. At this point, the nurse used a special machine that separated the sperm from the semen (I thought they were one and the same... but apparently, they are not). She then sucked the sperm into a long, thin syringe before directing me to go to the examination room to prepare.

I remember feeling calm while we were waiting for her. I felt good and I was very positive. I took my husband's hands in mine and I said I wanted to say a prayer. I am not a praying person, but I felt like this was one of the most important moments of our life, and there was no better time to ask God for help. We held each other's hands and asked for His help and to watch over us during this time. It's hard to explain, but the room felt blessed and holy.

The nurse came in and inserted the syringe past my cervix, right to where my eggs were. I could feel the pressure of the injection and tried to stay as still as possible. I remember she told me to breathe because I was holding my breath. When she was finished, she said I had to lie there for thirty minutes and just relax. I stayed still. In my mind, I felt like I could feel the sperm swimming and trying to find the egg. I was scared to move, thinking that I was going to disrupt its path.

Eventually, it was time to go and the waiting game began. We had to wait sixteen days before we could take a pregnancy test. And let me tell you, those were the longest days of my life. Especially the last few. I was so anxious. I couldn't think straight. It was the only thing on my mind. I couldn't focus on any conversation I was having with friends or family. My mind was 100% on what was going on inside of me. My poor family having to put up with me. I must have gone to the washroom ten times every hour. It's incredible the way the mind works. I constantly felt like I was getting my period. I remember going to the washroom just to wipe. Just to see if there was blood. It was exhausting. I only had one focus and that was on my body and waiting for any feeling or sign that I was pregnant.

Finally, the day fifteen came, and I hadn't gotten my period. I remember going to bed feeling very anxious and nervous. My periods were usually bang on, and now I was two days late. The feeling of hope that fills you is so immense. My chest was heavy, and I just wanted to fall asleep so that I could see what would happen the next morning.

I remember waking up and grabbing a tissue from the side of the bed. I wiped but I was scared to look. When I eventually glanced down, it was clean! No blood. I lay there, hopeful and scared at the same time. Could this really be happening? Please God let me be pregnant and I will never ask for anything again!

I remember that morning so well because the stillness in the room felt almost holy. The best way I can describe how I remember it was the feeling I had as a child on Christmas morning. When you are in bed and excited to see if Santa Clause came and all the magic that will come once your feet hit the floor.

When I took the pregnancy test and there were two lines I remember screaming with so much joy the whole neighborhood heard and I almost fell off the toilet!

Looking back, I should have held onto that feeling as long as I could, because it would be the only time I would ever see two lines on a pregnancy test

When my son was six months old and my period came back, we wanted to get right to it again. The early mornings at the clinic began again, this time with a child in tow. My mind was distracted as it felt less of an all or nothing situation. I am a big believer in mind over matter and I blame myself for being unfocused when I was there. During that time, my husband's job changed, and he wasn't able to be at the clinic like before. He was having to do his part at home, and I had to take the container of semen to the clinic. I always wondered if perhaps the journey from our house to the clinic took too long.

I remember sitting alone in our apartment one night. My husband was away for work and I had my 6th negative pregnancy test. We had absolutely no more money to spend on these procedures. I was so depressed, and I couldn't stop crying. I felt so trapped. I couldn't believe it was going to be money that was stopped us from having another child. In desperation, I called my mother late one night and asked to borrow money. She hesitated because of our six failed attempts. I exploded with anger, as I was stressed and very much feeling sorry for myself. I was mentally in a very dark place and my mother knew it. She didn't have problems lending us the money, she just didn't want me to continuously be disappointed. I didn't care about any of that. I only had a one-track mind and that to get pregnant again. In the end, my mom helped pay for two more attempts. Both failed.

On the 8th single lined pregnancy test, I sat on the edge of my bed, tears streaming down my face. Exhausted at all the wasted morning ultrasound visits.

Emotional from all the hormones I was taking.

Sore from injecting myself with needles.

Tired from all the times I held my breath and my prayers not being answered.

And totally depressed from the massive weight gain that happened, along with the depletion of all our money, which meant my husband and I had to declare bankruptcy.

I was mad at the world. Everything seemed unfair. And I felt like *no one* could understand what I was feeling. I was extremely vulnerable because when I was hopeful and everything went well and easy the first time, I was sharing my journey with everyone. But as I continued failing, I began to tell fewer and fewer people, and keeping everything inside felt very isolating. You feel like the only person in the world going through this. And when you tell your family and friends each time you have a negative result, it also becomes harder and harder for them to come up with something positive to say. You feel like you are in a lose-lose situation.

When I get depressed I have a tendency to become self-destructive, and I remember sitting on the bed and feeling so much anguish that I began pulling my hair and screaming. I loathed myself, my body, and my inadequacies as a woman. Having to tell my husband that the test was negative again.

And just when my self-sabotaging is at its worst, my three-year-old walked into see what was going on and if I was okay.

My heart stopped. He looked at me and put his little precious hand on my leg, and with his other hand, he touched the tears on my face. It was at that exact moment that something shifted in me. I remember it like it was yesterday. I looked at this miracle in front of me. My first attempt. The one that was to be. The one that God had chosen for me. He was mine and I was his. And that was it. Plain and simple. I didn't need anything more, and neither did he. This was how it was supposed to be.

It was time to STOP. It was time to appreciate this miracle that I was given, and it was time to be happy with everything I had. I had to stop looking for what was to come. For what was around the corner. Imagining a child that was never to be, while missing the child that I had right in front of me.

Looking back, I see that I needed to go down the path of eight negatives. I needed to have my son walk in and see me at my lowest self. Even though he was only three, at the time, he seemed so much wiser than me.

He is now ten years old, and they have been the best ten years of my life. After that moment we shared, everything changed. It was such a relief to be finished with trying. To have made the decision to stop. It felt like I had taken the heaviest shackles off, and it wasn't until they were off that I actually felt the weight of them. I was free. Free to live and pursue life, my life... *all* of it, not just one aspect. I began to mother without guilt. To feel content at having an only child and not feeling like I was letting him down.

And yes, there are days when he asks for a little brother or sister. And when this happens I go back to that place...but only for a few seconds because I realize that I have given him everything he has ever needed or wanted in life but this is something that he will have to live without. He will never have the experience of having siblings. He will be alone to navigate his role in our house. And because of this, we have grown his network in other ways. Making sure his life is full of friends and family. And I see that he is content. He is happy.

We adapt.

We accept.

We make the best of what we have.

I see this in him. When he comes home from friends that have lots of kids in the house, I see him happy to be home to a more quiet and simple life. I see him unwind as he appreciates what he has. This is when I know that as time goes by whether we are the parent or the child, we are given what we can handle. I've learned that we may have a plan for our life, but life has its own plans.

I now realize that I wasn't meant to have four children. One is plenty for us as a family. It works and it's good. Nothing is missing. We are a whole unit and the love is immense. And I look forward to every day.

Remember, science is a partner, not an enemy. If you cannot conceive naturally, don't look at it as a failure. Look at it as an intentional process that opens your eyes to how your body functions. Keeping you in tune with all the little feelings and emotions. Allowing you to be an active part in what will hopefully be the creation of the little love bug you have been praying for.

It may take longer.

It may feel unfair.

But it is your journey. And no one can take that away from you.

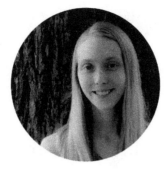

Sara Speicher

Sara Speicher is a wife and mother living in Western Pennsylvania. Shortly after graduating from Geneva College with her Bachelor's degree in Engineering, she married her husband and embarked on an adventure, moving twelve hours from their families to New Hampshire. There, Sara explored educational opportunities in child development and engaged in her new community, and she was blessed with her first son. After two years, her family moved back to Western Pennsylvania where Sara spends her days loving on her sweet toddler and looking for the path that God will lead her down next.

Connect with Sara:
speichersb1@gmail.com

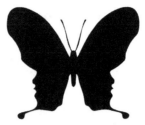

Rocked into Heaven's Arms

By Sara Speicher

My husband and I got married straight out of college. To celebrate our first wedding anniversary, we had a two-week-old baby boy, Z. My pregnancy with him had been as routine as it gets, with a thirty-nine-week delivery to a healthy baby boy. Before my husband and I got married, we had discussed having a large family of around five children, and we were off to a great start.

When Z was about to turn one, we started trying for another baby. While I did end up pregnant, we lost that baby to miscarriage at ten weeks gestation. I was devastated. I spent a full month in a very dark and deep depression. I didn't want anything to do with anybody during that time. Many people didn't even know I was pregnant, so I didn't want to then announce to people that my baby was gone. Our miscarriage occurred on June 30th, so on August 1st, I realized that I had 'lost' the whole month of July to my depression. I started trying to see people again and we also considered trying again for another baby. I didn't want to replace the baby that I had lost, but I still really wanted another baby. I have always wanted my children to be close together in age so that they would, hopefully, be good friends and playmates.

On September 21st, we learned that we were indeed expecting again, due near Z's second birthday. As long as I didn't miscarry this time, our babies would be exactly two years apart. I was very excited, but also very nervous about miscarrying again.

When I miscarried before, I started spotting about six weeks into the pregnancy until I miscarried. At six weeks into this pregnancy, I started spotting again. I was afraid, I was frustrated, and I felt like I was being mocked. I felt like I was going to lose my baby again. At nine weeks, we had an ultrasound and there was no more sign of the bleeding and a healthy little baby was growing inside me. I was shocked, but so thankful. From nine weeks until twelve weeks, everything seemed to be going well, so we made our big family announcements at twelve weeks over the Thanksgiving weekend.

At fourteen weeks, I was lying on the couch watching a movie with Z when I felt a gush. I didn't know what had happened, so I ran to the bathroom to discover blood was pouring out of me. My husband came home from work to take me to the emergency room. I thought it was obvious that the baby was gone, but the hospital did another ultrasound and the baby was kicking around and seemed to be fine. A strange peace came over me that this wasn't the end of our journey together. I was diagnosed with a subchorionic hematoma, which is a blood clot in the uterus that was partially behind the placenta. The doctor in the ER told me to prepare to miscarry and sent me home.

I called my OBGYN and told them what the ER doctor had said. They reassured me that, that subchorionic hematomas do happen, but miscarriage was by no means definite and there was still hope. I rested in that reassurance.

Over the weeks that followed, I continued to have spotting. My baby kept growing and we kept moving forward. It looked hopeful that we might be okay. When I reached twenty weeks, everything came crashing down on me once again. I started bleeding, heavily, daily, and would continue to do so for the remainder of the pregnancy. I was bleeding so much that the doctors were concerned that I was going to bleed to death. Many of my doctors strongly encouraged me to consider an abortion, because if I didn't, I was going to die. My baby boy was alive and kicking and worth fighting for. I knew I had a husband and another son who needed me, but I couldn't kill the living, moving son in my womb.

This was also the time that I had my anatomy scan. Our son had lots of markers that suggested he was going to have a genetic disorder. Even if most of the markers turned out to be nothing, he definitely had a heart defect. More doctors sat down with me and advised me to have an abortion. They couldn't understand that my son was worth fighting for. They said things like, "You are young and healthy, so you should just end this pregnancy and start again," and, "don't you know all the problems this baby has? You don't want to deal with that." They reminded me over and over again that my baby wasn't perfect, I was young, and I was going to die. They couldn't change my mind; I wasn't going to kill him.

The bleeding continued to get worse and my blood count continued to drop. I was admitted to the hospital for the last three weeks of my pregnancy for very close monitoring. The doctors gave me many interventions to try to boost baby as best we could and prepare for an early delivery. When my water broke at only twenty-five weeks, it was only a matter of time before my son would have to be born.

My time in the hospital was really hard on me and my family. My husband had to keep working and my toddler had to move in with my mother since I could not care for him. My family was torn in three different directions and we were all feeling the pain of that. The doctors kept taking away my regular diet in place of an all-liquid diet because there were many days they thought we were heading for an emergency C-section. I weighed less when my son was born than when I got pregnant with him, and I am naturally petite.

For five days I was having contractions and the bleeding was so heavy that the doctors determined that my placenta was no longer doing its job well enough. As a result, my son and I would be in worse shape in a week than we were that day. At twenty-seven-and-a-half weeks, they induced me. We knew the risks of having a baby so premature, but we made it two months further than the doctors thought possible. In an attempt to now save both of our lives, it was time for our baby boy to come. It was a short and easy labor. He took his first breath and let out a cry on his own. At two pounds four ounces, our sweet baby Anthony was here! I was so relieved.

I was so thankful that he cried on his own and seemed to be doing well for such a tiny baby. I was so thankful that I could finally start to heal after months and months of heavy bleeding. I had not realized just how much physical pain I had been in until after he was born. My pain disappeared so quickly that I felt better within a day. Now we could focus on him and not me. We knew I was okay now. Now we just needed to get our baby boy bigger and stronger so our family could be united once again.

I was released from the hospital when Anthony was a day and a half old and my husband and I headed straight over to the children's hospital he had been transferred to. We looked at our tiny little boy in the incubator covered in wires. I looked at his nurse who always had a warm smile on her face. She told me that she loved Anthony and he was her only buddy for the day. Sometimes they had two babies assigned to a nurse. If the only thing the babies needed was time to grow, they would have three babies, but Anthony needed the extra attention and she was honored to be his nurse.

They performed ultrasounds on Anthony to see how he was doing. His heart was exactly how they expected it to be. He needed surgery for him to be able to live outside of the NICU, but he had to be roughly five pounds with no other complications to be able to have that surgery. They did an ultrasound on his head because some preemies have brain bleeds from being so small. When he was in the same hospital I was, he had a small brain bleed on one hemisphere of his brain. Now that he was in the children's hospital, he also had a larger bleed on the other side of his brain. The doctors told us that he may have a variety of developmental delays and possibly even seizures. There is nothing that can be done for brain tissue that has had blood pooled on it. All we could do was see if it would stop from getting worse and work with what we had.

After three weeks in the hospital, I wanted a night in a normal bed, so I went to my mother's house and got to give Z a hug for the first time in weeks. I cried looking at him. He was still so tiny himself. Why had I rushed into a second baby when my first baby was still so tiny? I knew things didn't look good for Anthony and I knew if he stayed in the NICU I would be torn between my babies for a long, long time. Z and I cried together. He stroked my hair as the tears ran quickly down both of our cheeks.

I slept in the next day out of pure exhaustion and was woken up to go back to the hospital around lunchtime. We were not prepared for the news that we would get. Not only had Anthony's brain not stopped bleeding, but the bleeding had gotten so severe that one hemisphere of his brain was now crushing the other, and blood was pooling at the base of his brain. He was only breathing because the machine did it for him. His heart was only beating because a machine did it for him. His body temperature and everything else only looked like he was doing well because of machines. The doctors told us that his condition could not be improved. There was nothing that could be done to help him. At some point, the blood would pool enough that even the machines couldn't keep him 'alive' anymore. They could keep him in that state until it happened. Even if he stopped bleeding, the damage was already done. He would never be free of all of the machines.

My heart broke. My baby wasn't really living. I imagine he was hurting. I couldn't let him 'live' like that. I wouldn't want to live like that. I believe in a good and loving God that would welcome my sweet boy into His heaven. With heavy hearts, we asked if we could hold him. We weren't able to up to that point since he hadn't been stable enough. We asked if we could take pictures with him. We asked if Z could come into the NICU and take pictures with Anthony so we would have a picture of us as a family of four. The doctors and nurses were so loving and willing to accommodate. At 6:48 pm, the same time he entered this world, we took all his tubes away. We sang to him and held him and rocked him.

My son was a fighter. I will forever be convinced that if his brain hadn't bled, his heart would have been fine. We were told when the tubes came off him he may hold on for a couple of minutes or a couple of hours, but there was no way to know. He fought for two and a half hours before he took his last breath and his heartbeat for the last time in my arms. The whole time we held him, we sang worship songs to him. We told him about Jesus and the Heaven that was waiting for him, and that someday mommy and daddy and Anthony would all be reunited again. We told him how thankful we were for him, how much we loved him, and that we didn't want him to hurt anymore. "It's okay baby. Let go. Go to Jesus. It's okay. We love you so so so much." We prayed and asked God to sweep him up into Heaven's arms.

Finally, he left us. I didn't want him to have to go, but I so badly wanted to know that his pain and suffering were gone and that he was whole and safe in the arms of Jesus.

We left the hospital that night empty-handed and exhausted, happy, and sad. Happy for his suffering to be over. Sad that he couldn't be home with us and grow up with his big brother. Sad that the two of them weren't going to get into all kinds of mischief together. Sad, that my dream of my two close buddies was crushed.

I had fought and fought and fought for him. I was ready to give my own life for him if it could have saved him. At the end of it all, God is the giver of life and He knows the number of our days. Psalm 139:16 says, "Your eyes saw my unformed body; all the days ordained for me were written in your book before one of them came to be." (NIV) Anthony had three days. He was so loved during those three days and *always* will be loved. We are thankful for the time we were given with Anthony and will treasure our memories with him forever, though they are few.

But now? After everything I went through, was it worth it? If he was going to die no matter what, and, if I had known that, would I have made a different choice? Would I have ended his life eight weeks sooner in the womb-like the doctors told me to? Not a chance. Why? Because he was worth it. The name Anthony means priceless, and he is. He is priceless. He has been worth every pain and every tear and always will be. Why? Because I am thankful to be his mommy. I am thankful that God gave him to me to watch over and to care for and to love. Anthony changed me and brought me so much joy in his short life. I know there are other mommies out there who wish someone understood what it was like to go through a hard and trying pregnancy and still not get to bring their baby home. I know there are mommies that have had preemie babies who were left in the NICU very small and fragile. I know there are mommies out there who need to know that they are not alone! Because I have felt alone. I've met people who have had miscarriages, and stillborns, and their stories break my heart! However, I have met so few who have rocked their young, young baby into Heaven's arms like I did.

Every baby's life matters and always will matter, regardless of how short their life is or how many extra needs they may have.

God makes every mama and every baby for a reason and He doesn't make mistakes. God's heart breaks for you as you are in pain and crying, because He loves you. You will love your baby forever and hold their memory dear to your heart. Even as others forget and move on you know you will never stop loving and remembering them.

I know and believe all these things to be true, and yet, this road has not been easy. A month after our son died I started having extreme anxiety and panic attacks. I felt like I was going to die. For all of my effort, I could not regain control of myself. I have lost my appetite and have lost a lot of weight, weighing less than 100 lbs. for the first time since middle school. I have days where I cry a lot and days my body just physically aches from my loss.

I've learned a lot more about grief than I ever have before. I see now how harmful suppressing your emotions is and how important it is to take the time to grieve. Don't suppress your emotions. Take time to grieve. I have been told I will always grieve, but it will get better and I will be able to better function again someday.

Taking the time to remember Anthony and to cry because of how much I love him and miss him has been very cathartic for me. Ever so slowly, my body and my mind and my soul are being healed and restored as I lean into Jesus. Of course I have had many setbacks along the way. My due date was an incredibly hard day, knowing that was when he should have arrived and I should have a newborn at home. I also had several friends and family members have healthy May and June babies and mine is missing. It is a long road with many bumps. I have been forced to slow down and be thankful for what I do have and also wonder about the path God has still in store for me. After all, He could have let me die in my pregnancy with Anthony, but He sustained me. I know He's not done with me yet. I don't know what He has planned, but I know there is a plan and it is good.

I truly wish that I had an amazing and encouraging conclusion to my story. I wish I could say, "But I went on to have four more beautiful healthy babies with no complications". However, my story is still being written. Anthony was born and died in March 2019, and I am still in the thick of recovery. I don't know if there are more babies in my future. I don't know if I will have many more losses, many more births, or no more pregnancies. I don't know if we will adopt any children or have any more biological children. I don't know if Z will now remain an 'only' child, because of the brother he never got to grow up with. I don't have a conclusion to my story to give you hope. But I do have hope. I have hope that Anthony will bless many with his short time on earth. I have faith that God knows how many total children He will ever give me and that number may just be the three I have already had or it may be many more.

I have had many people approach me and tell me how strong I am because of how I've handled my pregnancy and my loss of Anthony. I don't feel strong. In fact, I feel very weak. It is only through God's strength that I can continue to carry on each and every day. "But he said to me, "My grace is sufficient for you, for my power is made perfect in weakness." Therefore, I will boast all the more gladly about my weaknesses, so that Christ's power may rest on me. That is why, for Christ's sake, I delight in weaknesses, in insults, in hardships, in persecutions, in difficulties. For when I am weak, then I am strong." (2 Corinthians 12:9-10, NIV)

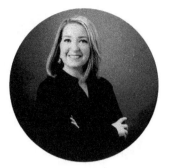

Leslie Tremblay

Leslie Tremblay, originally from British Columbia, Canada, resides in Alberta, Canada with her husband, son, and puppy.

Leslie's ambition and education have been her pathway to achieving a rewarding career in team leadership and professional administrator roles. She is a lifelong learner with an ongoing desire to investigate the more intrinsic qualities in life and what makes us who we become.

She continuously steps outside her comfort zone, both personally and professionally, knowing that this is the only way one grows. Her passions include family, travel, community service and inspiring and empowering others to become better versions of themselves through guidance in personal and professional advancement/ development.

Leslie is a best-selling author and her life is about balance and not giving up on her dreams.

Connect with Leslie:
https://www.instagram.com/tremblay_leslie/
https://www.facebook.com/leslietremblayauthor/

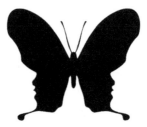

Darkness to Light: The Courage to Share

By Leslie Tremblay

The universe has a funny way of guiding us in directions that we had never imagined. One truth that I've come to know and trust is that the universe has the best of intentions in mind. We're the ones that get in our own way.

I had never intended on telling this story... ever. Up to the point of committing to putting pen to paper to write in this book, only a handful of people knew bits and pieces of my journey, and only one knows it all. That person is Frederic, my love and my partner in this journey.

The decision to share was difficult. My mind was saying, *Please stop, protect yourself. You're being too vulnerable.* My heart, however, spoke softly, almost a whisper. *You need to do this, it's time.* I listened to my heart and here I am.

My greatest hope is that my story will inspire or empower you in some way big or small. You are not alone.

What tough decision have you made lately?

You may be asking yourself, why now? What was my motivation to share?

Simply put, I let the 'cat-out-of-the-bag' to help an amazing passion project, *Footprints: Infertility & Pregnancy Loss Support Group*, headed up by a friend and fellow author/speaker Blaise Hunter. Her passion lit a flicker in me that turned into a flame, and I wanted to share a tidbit to help with fundraising efforts for her non-profit support group. A group I had wished existed as I drifted through my own grueling journey. I started with a social media post that led to a connection that, well…led me to Danielle, our amazing book compiler. Remember what I said about the universe guiding us? It won't always be a loud resounding clatter, but sometimes a simple soft whisper.

What is being whispered to you?

Don't let fear hold you back, lean into that fear and find out what is really going on. You never know what's around the corner for you or when an opportunity will present itself.

The Day I'll Never Forget

"I'm sorry, there's no heartbeat. Your doctor is expecting you."

Wait… what?

That moment will stay with me for as long as I live and breathe. Silence and disbelief washed over me and all I could do is just stand there, motionless. I was in my blue hospital gown and all I could do is look at Frederic. Little did I know at that moment; that would be the start of the most gut-wrenching journey I'd ever taken. Sure, I've had struggles, obstacles, and immense heartbreak but this… this was a doozy.

Did you have this experience? What was your experience? What was it like for you?

Take my hand and walk with me through this journey… please hold on tight. We will get through this together.

It's So Unfair

The most commonly asked question during my fourteen-years of marriage was, "So when are you going to have children?" I came to detest this question. It's not like we weren't trying. We did want children, but hadn't been successful in our pursuit. I didn't appreciate the constant reminder. I finally got to the point of saying, "Please stop asking." They eventually did.

Every month that passed with a negative test was draining to my spirit. I would often see stories of children being harmed or neglected and I would get angry, asking, *Why? Why did these people get the privilege of having children and I couldn't?* So unfair.

Our marriage did not survive. Not solely because we couldn't become parents together, but it did play a part, whether we wanted to admit it or not. We drifted apart and neither one of us put in the effort trying to keep it going. We cared for each other but were no longer in love with each other. We called it quits—he went his way and I went mine.

He met someone, fell in love, got married and she became pregnant. How do you think I was feeling at that moment? Well, I'll tell you…. broken. Utterly broken. I was convinced it was my fault that we couldn't have children. In some way I was defective, doomed to a barren life.

Our mind plays tricks on us sometimes. Thoughts of being the crazy cat lady passed through my mind on several occasions. At least I did have a good head start, as I already had two cats. With Winston and Junior by my side, it was us against the world. They were incredible companions, there to give me loads of love, and I gave it back.

Light After Dark

A few years after my divorce, I met my handsome Frederic. Conversations around children did come up and I was completely honest with him. I filled him in on my story and told him I didn't think that I could have kids. This was one of those crucial conversations that would make or break us. We decided that I should get some tests done to see if there was a medical problem that could be treated. I was still convinced that I was broken.

During our consult, we were encouraged to try while I awaited my referral to the specialist. My consult was in July and my referral was made for December.

Any guesses as to what happened during that time?

You guessed it! I became pregnant in August but didn't catch on until October—eight weeks later. *Crazy!* I wasn't broken and barren after all, I just didn't have the right combination the first time. I was one of the fortunate ones who had an amazing pregnancy, the only time I got sick was during the C-section. He didn't want to come out, so they had to go in and get him.

At the age of forty-two, I became a mom for the first time.

Together, we decided that I would go back to work after three months and Frederic would take the remainder of the year as paternity leave. He had a fantastic leave program. We thought this was a great plan and still stand firm on it today, but boy-oh-boy, there was judgment all around for this decision, and most surprisingly, it came from women. The men thought Frederic was a rock star saying, "Wow this is great, I could never do that," and he received many pats on the back. I, however, was met with, "I don't know how you can do that," "I would never be able to leave my child," and "I would miss them too much." I'm sure they weren't trying to hurt my feelings, but it felt like backhanded compliments with an implied undertone of, how could you leave your baby? I'd give my life for my little man. Me going back to work was never about not loving him enough, we felt it was the best decision for our family. Frederic is an incredibly capable man and a great father. I always felt and still feel like I must defend that, but to be honest, between the two of us, he makes the better stay at home parent. I used to feel guilty, but I don't anymore. Older and wiser perhaps.

We had talked about having another baby, and were actively trying, but there was no pressure. If it happened it happened. I mean, I had Dominic when I was forty-two and was now forty-four, so time was not on our side.

Two Positives, Very Different Emotions

In November 2016, amid home renovations, I realized I was late. Off to the pharmacy I went to get a pregnancy test.

It was positive!

Just to be sure, I made an appointment with my doctor that same day. It was a quick visit to tell him my pregnancy test came back positive and I wanted to verify the results. He happily gave me the requisitions to do that. As I hadn't been there in a while, he also ordered some general blood work and a couple of other tests.

I anxiously awaited the official results to come in but needed to wait over the weekend to hear back. Sure enough, I was pregnant. Dominic was going to be a big brother! I was referred to the same prenatal clinic as my first pregnancy in a nearby community and I would see them at the end of the week. Due to my age, I was expecting to be there more often than usual.

The happy feelings soon faded as I was called back to my doctor's office two days later with results from the other tests that were performed. The results were not so good. One of the tests was a cancer pre-screen that came back positive. Two positive tests with a very different set of emotions. More tests of a different nature were in order.

Sitting in the car, I called my husband and told him he needed to come home. I managed to get myself home before he got there, and then I completely lost it. Barely able to speak, I handed him my results. The words, "What are we going to do?" was all I could whisper.

Two days later came my appointment at the prenatal clinic. I had to explain the positive cancer pre-screen results and asked what needed to happen next. I was a mess, and they were very kind and patient with me. This was supposed to be a happy time. I was not happy. I wanted to get the additional testing done that would require a procedure, they wouldn't do it while I was pregnant, and I would have to wait until the baby was born. This upset me even further.

"First things first, let's check on the baby," said my doctor. He performed his exam, feeling around, listening for a heartbeat, etc. I didn't think anything of it at the time, but he didn't offer to let me hear the heartbeat. Did he know at that time? Again because of my age, I was sent for a twelve-week ultrasound a few weeks later.

It was a few days before Christmas when the ultrasound day finally arrived. I had been feeling better and coming to terms with the possible cancer diagnosis, but was looking forward to seeing my baby. The technician started the exam, and this time, I couldn't see the screen. I was at a different angle, but I thought, *No matter, eventually she'll let me see and hear the heartbeat.*

During the exam, she excused herself for a little while. I don't even remember why she told me she was leaving. She asked if my husband was with me. I said yes and then asked for him to come in. So, he did. This was standard procedure at the time, I was the only one allowed in the room during the initial exam. We were standing there, and the words came out. "I'm sorry, there's no heartbeat. Your doctor is expecting you." Then off she went. Stunned with what we just heard, I got dressed and we left in silence.

We got into the car. I looked at him, started to cry and said, "I'm so sorry." Self-blame was settling in. *This was all my fault. I've caused this to happen.*

The prenatal clinic was a long, thirty-five-minute car ride away. We arrived, I pulled myself together, and we walked into the clinic side-by-side, avoiding eye contact with anyone. I had to wait in line and then tell the receptionist why I was there. I had a complete meltdown and could barely get the words out. I stood off to the side in a corner, not looking at anyone. One of the nurses came to get us and escorted us into a tiny exam room to await the doctor's arrival.

After what felt like an eternity, the doctor arrived. She was kind and sympathetic and gave us the cold hard facts: you can take these pills or let it pass on its own. That was a tough on-the-spot decision to have to make, but we made it together. We opted for the pills.

We went to the pharmacy and I really was doing my best to hold myself together, but she asked the question, "Are you pregnant?" I went into meltdown mode again and responded, "I *was*," before she whisked us off to the consult room.

Frederic was with me the entire time. You may be asking yourself, why didn't he do the talking? Well you see, I'm very stubborn, but at least I know it. I forgot that he suffered a loss too but honestly, I could only think about myself at that moment. The pharmacist filled the Rx and explained what needed to be done before we headed home. Frederic dropped me off, got me settled and went to pick Dominic up from daycare. He really is amazing.

I did my best to keep my composure, but in reality, was just trying not to fall apart for the rest of the night because I still needed to be a mom and didn't want my son to see me in a mess. He wouldn't understand. We carried on with our evening the best we could until Dominic was in bed. We made all the necessary phone calls, there weren't many as we had decided to wait until after the ultrasound to make it public. I'm glad we made that decision.

We sat together and read through our instructions copied on a simple white piece of paper. Reality setting in, we discussed what now needed to happen, and how we would do it together. The instructions explained how to use the medication and what to expect.

They write about bleeding out, so I lined the bed with a plastic picnic tablecloth just in case. Frederic was there with me and he inserted the medication. He cried. I cried and apologized. I had to lie on my back for an hour. The room was dark, cool and silent. Several thoughts raced through my head. *How did this happen? Did I stress myself out too much because of the positive cancer screen and cause this?* I felt like a complete failure.

The process was repeated for two nights until Dec 24th. We had planned on staying home for Christmas, but I just couldn't do it. I didn't want to be at home. I'm not a fan of winter travel but we immediately made plans to leave the next day to head out on a six-hour drive to my moms to spend the rest of our Christmas vacation.

We're Not Done Yet

The bleeding was quite heavy, more than a normal period but that's what I expected. We got through Christmas well and into early January.

One beautiful, surprisingly mild winter day, we decided to do some pre-spring-cleaning during Dominic's nap, and then it happened. I noticed that I was changing my pad frequently, much too often—and then the gushing came. I came out of the washroom and said, "Frederic you need to take me to the hospital." He is amazing in an emergency. He had Dominic out of bed and strapped in his car seat with a folded-up towel for me to sit on by the time I got to the truck.

Ten minutes later, I was in the emergency room, blood running down my legs, and proceeded directly to the nursing station where they took me in immediately.

Once again, I explained that I had a miscarriage and was hemorrhaging. They brought me into a private exam room and gave me a gown to wear. I was physically a mess. When the doctor arrived the first thing she said was, "Why didn't they take you directly to the OR?" I obviously didn't have an answer to that one. Then came the internal exam. Wow, that was painful. She kept telling me to relax. *Really? Relax? Well, I'll do my best.* I was surprised to hear the words, "There is still a lot of product left." Product is what they use to reference the fetus. During the exam, I explained that we were told we lost the baby at seven to eight weeks.

Once again, words I won't forget: "By the size of it, I would say you were further along."

OMG, what? Did they make a mistake on the ultrasound? Seriously?

What followed for the next few hours were meds to stop the bleeding and subsequent internal exams until I was finally able to go home later that evening.

Prior to leaving, I was given a requisition for yet another ultrasound to see if all the 'product' had been released. Thankfully, I got in quickly only to discover there was still some hanging on.

I went back to the clinic and met with the OBGYN who confirmed that I needed a D&C, which they scheduled for the next morning.

Morning came. We dropped Dominic off at daycare and off we went to the hospital. I do have to say the nurses were great. I was walking down the hall to the surgery room when one of the doctors asked, "How much blood do you think you lost? You are looking pale and your counts are low. There is a possibility that you will need a blood transfusion." *Enough already!* I said to myself.

The D&C went smoothly from what I was told, and thankfully no transfusion was required, but I did need to take iron supplements for many weeks after.

Getting Back to 'Normal'... Sort Of

I spent the next couple of weeks recovering physically and mentally before heading back to work full time. As I mentioned previously, I didn't tell many people I was pregnant, so when I went back, I didn't have to talk about what happened. My team just thought I had taken some last-minute vacation time.

Now that the painful part was over, my next challenge was getting the additional testing done due to the positive cancer pre-screen that they refused to do while I was pregnant. I had to wait until my iron levels were back up before they would proceed.

Weeks later I had a colonoscopy and was told that everything was good. No cancer. I was so thankful for this positive result.

This entire ordeal was difficult, and it will stay with me forever. However, I have been able to move through it positively. It did take hard work and time for me to stop blaming myself. If it was meant to be it would have been. Mindset shifts were the most important aspect of my healing, I couldn't change what happened, but I could come out the other side as a better person.

Dominic still asks for a sister every now and then. Although we haven't be able to give him what he's asked for, we did give him the next best thing, a female puppy named Lylas. They are best friends; it's a love hate relationship.

Dominic is my little miracle and I'm so grateful for the opportunity to be his mom. Our job is to teach him well and help him to be the best person he can be.

As mentioned at the beginning of my story, I hadn't intended to ever put pen to paper and tell my story. I left out the graphic gory details, as anyone who's gone through this experience knows. My intention in sharing my story is to provide hope and inspiration. I became a first-time mom at the age of forty-two to a magnificent little man. We haven't been successful on the sibling front but have tried to convince Frederic's younger brother and his wife to have lots of kids, so he'll at least have lots of cousins. We'll see how that goes.

The journey of grief and loss can be devastating but you have to believe that you will be okay. It will take some time. You may never be the same and perspectives will change however, use your energy for good: seek support and be that support. Someone else needs you.

There is life after loss and you will breathe again, I promise you that.

Stories and books like this are necessary. They need to be read and promoted to help one another heal. You are not alone.

My Biggest Lesson

Gratitude is the greatest lesson here.

I am grateful for my son Dominic.

I am grateful for my love Frederic.

I am grateful for my family and friends.

I am grateful for the lessons learned in becoming a mom.

Everyone has a history.
What you do with it is up to you.
Some repeat it.
Some learn from it.
The really special ones use it to help others.

~ JM Green

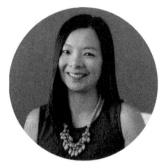

Adrienne Wei, L.Ac

Adrienne Wei is a multi-passionate entrepreneur and integrative fertility guru living in Charlotte, North Carolina.

After realizing Corporate America was not her cup of tea, Adrienne decided to follow her mother's footsteps to become a doctor in Chinese medicine. Fueled by personal passion, education, and advocacy, Adrienne has dedicated her career to helping women everywhere become mothers.

Adrienne is a board-certified fertility acupuncture specialist and creator of Practically Fertile™ Methodology for fertility and hormone balance. Adding to her accolades, Adrienne is a fellow of the American Board of Oriental Reproductive Medicine (ABORM) and also board certified in Chinese herbology by the National Certification Commission for Acupuncture and Oriental Medicine (NCCAOM).

Her experienced all-female team continues to make a deep impact in the lives of women who are trying-to-conceive. Globally, her trademarked methodology reaches thousands of women who turn to her for answers.

When she is not busy helping women get pregnant, Adrienne is a loving wife and a proud mother.

Connect with Adrienne:
www.practicallyfertileclub.com
www.ipacupuncture.com
www.adriennewei.com

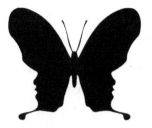

We Are Not Broken

By Adrienne Wei, L.Ac

Unlike many of you, I have not experienced the loss of a precious pregnancy. Instead, I want to tell you about self-advocacy and how I successfully overcame polycystic ovarian syndrome (PCOS), which then led to the discovery of a passion for helping others.

I remember the exact moment when my gynecologist, who was a man, looked at me and said, "You have what we call polycystic ovarian syndrome or PCOS."

I remember this moment so vividly because of the rush of emotions that came after. I was confused... *What the heck is PCOS, I've never heard of this before.* I felt ashamed... *I must have done something to my body that caused this, I'm a screw up, I must keep this a secret.* I felt scared ... *What if this means I can never get pregnant, what would my future husband think?*

I asked my doctor, "How did I end up with this condition?"

He said, "I don't know, we don't understand everything about this condition yet. You have extremely irregular cycles, you have cysts on the ovaries, it is what it is."

I then asked the question I was afraid to get the answer to: "Does this mean I won't be able to get pregnant in the future?"

"I'm not sure," he said. "Maybe... maybe not... but in the meantime, you can take birth control pills and see what happens."

Birth control pills... the very thing you take to *prevent* a pregnancy. I was told to take the pill and wait and see, and *maybe* the PCOS wouldn't affect my chances of becoming a mother later.

I walked out of his office in a weird state of mind. I can't fully explain how I felt. There was relief, knowing there was a reason why I didn't get my periods on a regular basis but also anxiety, because the only way to correct the condition was to take medicine.

I wanted to meet the man of my dreams, get married, and become a mother. What would happen if the problem returned after I stopped taking them?

I felt at a loss. I didn't have answers, and I didn't know what the future would bring.

Let me backtrack a bit and just say that up until that point, I had next to no education about the female reproductive system besides what was taught in biology and health classes. I spent the first eleven years of my life in a country (China) with a culture that saw sex as dirty (I'm talking about the 'old' China, not the modernized China).

TV programs and books were censored and there were *zero* discussions about sex at school and at home... it was a taboo subject. There was also zero education about how our bodies functioned. It was believed that if we knew how our bodies worked, we would be more likely to have premarital sex.

I moved to the United States at the age of eleven and was thrown into a completely different world. The words 'culture shock' didn't truly describe this transition.

I was surprised that girls wore super low-cut shirts. Where I came from, you would get reprimanded for showing too much skin and you would bring shame to your family. I didn't know you could start dating as a teenager. Where I came from, you saved yourself for 'the one'. My parents have been together since they were sixteen.

I didn't know you could watch two people make out on primetime TV. Where I came from, even seeing a man and woman hug was enough to make someone blush.

I was one of the last girls in my grade to get her period. I was made fun of by other girls because what kind of weirdo doesn't have her period by the time she's ten!? When I finally got my period, I had no idea what was really happening. I came home with a stain on my underwear. Mom gave me a pad and showed me how to use it, and that was it.

I was really hoping for a hug from her, or a smile to tell me, "Hey you're a woman now." But my mom wasn't that kind of person. Looking back, it was a scary time of my life because I was venturing into the unknown.

No one explained to me that you get a period because it all starts in the brain, in the hypothalamus. There is this hormone called gonadotropin-releasing hormone (GnRH) that sends a signal every month to the pituitary gland.

Then there's a hormone called follicle-stimulating hormone (FSH) that comes from the Pituitary gland and stimulates the ovaries to produce follicles. Another hormone called estrogen helps the follicles to mature. When the follicles are ready, the luteinizing hormone (LH) causes one follicle to rupture and release an egg.

Afterward, the site where the follicle has just ruptured becomes what's called the corpus luteum which secretes progesterone. The progesterone thickens the uterine lining in preparation for pregnancy, and the lining sheds if there's no pregnancy. And *voila*! You get your period.

If there is a glitch during any of these steps, you're going to have problems with your cycle.

I'm thankful for all this knowledge nowadays, and I'm counting down the days when I can have this talk with my own daughter. I'm so excited to share with her what I have learned so that she can be educated about how her own body works.

So there I was, diagnosed with a condition that I didn't quite understand, and no one seemed to be able to provide any answers or solutions other than birth control pills.

If I had been a fan of birth control pills, I probably would have listened to the doctor and just taken them. However, I took them briefly for six months in college and it was the worst experience ever. I felt bloated all the time, I was moody, I was emotional, I didn't feel like myself. So, despite only getting my period a couple of times a year, I never wanted to take the pill. I knew most women got their periods every month, but no one said that not getting your period once a month *wasn't* normal either. So, I just let it be.

I felt kind of lost outside of the doctor's office. I walked home and the entire time I was thinking, *I am an idiot.* How could I have not known this? How could I let this go on for so long without doing something about it?

I was twenty-six years old at the time and in my second year of acupuncture school. And between you and me, honestly, I chose this career path initially because I didn't know what else to do with my life... a conversation for another day.

I wasn't ready to become a mom; I didn't even have a steady boyfriend. But when I knew I had a condition that could potentially derail my plans of starting a family later and I was studying Chinese medicine, I decided to experiment on myself. I decided that if it worked, I'd be ahead of the 8-ball. I'd be ready when I found my soulmate.

Chinese medicine has been around for three thousand years, so it must work, right? Where would the Chinese civilization be if it didn't? That was my logic.

I started by consulting with a clinic supervisor who specialized in women's health. Her reaction was not what I expected. She gasped and said, "What?! Oh my God, you have PCOS?" Right away I felt discouraged—like I might be wasting my time. Luckily, the next thing she said was, "Let's work on this together and regulate your cycle."

Whew! It is possible then to get rid of this thing, I thought to myself.

I started my acupuncture and herbal regimen that day.

For the next few years, I stuck to a regular acupuncture treatment routine. I tested different herbal formulas on myself based on classroom learnings and advice from different teachers at school. Some worked great, and some didn't. I soaked up every morsel of knowledge that I could find about PCOS. From books to blogs to research articles. I would come to learn that there are four-types of PCOS, who knew! And mine was considered a type four or 'Lean PCOS'. I would also learn that PCOS is heavily related to the hormone insulin, which means it can be reversed through diet and lifestyle changes alone.

No gynecologists I saw have ever suggested anything else that I could do besides take birth control pills. But I didn't care, because I was not going to take artificial hormones.

Slowly but steadily, my cycles became more regular. It was never twenty-eight days (FYI, only 15% of women have twenty-eight-day cycles) but I was getting more than three periods a year. I was amazed at how much better I was feeling overall. My skin has never looked better. My mood swings were minimal.

Unfortunately, I wasn't able to practice on someone else other than myself, because inside the student clinic, very few patients sought treatment for fertility-related issues. I thought to myself, *If only I knew other women who had this same condition. I could do so much to help them.*

I moved to Charlotte, North Caroline within two months of graduating from acupuncture school and opened my own clinic. I was excited and scared like anyone starting a brand new business.

I was still hoping to help other women overcome hormone imbalances, but like any new business, making money was a top priority. You couldn't be picky about who walked in through your doors and what they were seeking treatment for.

I truly believe the universe was watching out for me because I believed so strongly in what I wanted to do.

One day, a new patient named Shanna walked into my office in tears and told me that she was having trouble getting pregnant because she had PCOS. Within six weeks of working with Shanna, applying what I knew at the time about PCOS, she became pregnant! I lost count of the number of "thank you's" I got. I had never felt so accomplished. I couldn't believe that Chinese medicine worked for someone else other than myself. The fact that I helped her achieve a lifelong dream after everything else had failed her...the fact that I just helped to bring a human being into this world, I felt the universe was sending me some type of sign—nudging me.

A couple of days later, an older lady told me about her wish to have a baby. Within six weeks, she was pregnant too!

It was then that I discovered there was a common underlying theme. They'd exhausted all other options because they'd been told that there's something wrong with their bodies—that pregnancy wasn't possible without drastic measures.

I realized that so little education was available for those trying to get pregnant. Doctors don't take the time to explain anything because there is a pill for everything and most people are not taught to look at their bodies holistically. They don't know how to align the body and mind.

My mission became clear to me. This is what I was destined to do, to help other women become mothers.

I overcame my condition because I refused to listen to the doctors. This was my chance to educate and empower these women to start trusting their bodies again and start believing that a woman's body is amazing.

I've been dedicating my entire career to this mission since then.

In the meantime, I ended up meeting my best friend and soulmate, Nathaniel. We became pregnant right away after getting married. I don't say this to make anyone jealous or feel bad. I know we were very lucky that we didn't struggle.

I became pregnant because of the hard work I put in upfront to beat PCOS. I am my own success story. I am proof that you shouldn't always listen to your doctor. You always have options, even when you feel like there are none.

Today, I'm considered an integrative fertility expert in the community because of my vast knowledge and the integration of Chinese medicine and modern functional medicine into a trademarked methodology, Practically Fertile™.

To date, I have helped to bring almost one thousand Acu-babies into this world, with a little help from my team. A huge shout-out to the amazing women I work with every day.

We've helped women who were told pregnancy isn't possible without a donor egg to get pregnant on their own. We've helped women who have suffered five miscarriages to become pregnant and stay pregnant. We've helped women who were diagnosed with 'unexplained infertility' and thought IVF was the only option to become pregnant after tweaking a few things in their diet. My favorite success stories are those women with PCOS, whose cycles I helped regulate through diet and exercise alone.

My dear friend, we've never met. I don't know your name, I don't know where you are on your journey of trying-to-conceive, but I want to tell you this: I see you. No matter what anyone says. No matter what you have been told or what you have thought about yourself.

You are amazing. Your body is amazing. Trust that you already intuitively know what is best for you.

I wish you the best of luck on your journey wherever it might lead you.

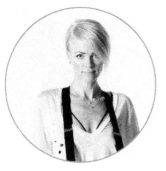

Shannon Wooten

Shannon Wooten is a life coach, writer, and author of the book, *Infertility Sucks, You Don't!*

She is an advocate for your healed struggle, and a visionary that will help you lead your life in a way that allows you to stop feeling held back and start living liberated. Shannon's focus is to bring the power of you to the surface. It is to reunite you with the natural energy inside begging to get out.

Shannon is unashamed to share that she has lived in the gutter of struggle, felt the pain of a dying self-confidence, and nearly lost who she was. She has rediscovered joy and emerged again, a dedicated and empowered woman who believes you are not lost in this and that you can find you, and your joy, again, too.

Connect with Shannon:
https://www.instagram.com/shannonwooten/
https://www.facebook.com/wootenshannon
http://www.lifewithshannon.com/

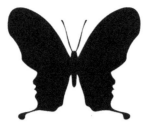

You Are Not Broken, You Are Being Built.

By Shannon Wooten

Walking from the doctor's office, each thundering step turned into ringing in my ears as the information sank in… "It may be difficult for you to conceive."

The ringing was loud and something I had *never* experienced before. It vibrated inside of me.

Just as quickly as it reverberated through my head, it stopped the blood flow to my face and seized all bodily movement. Luckily, by the time it hit me, I was within reach of my car door.

I stretched for the handle and collapsed into the driver's seat. I had no air. I didn't know where the oxygen went, but it had left me. With each expeditious inhale, exhale, I could feel the muscles in my chest thump harder and with more deliberateness.

I wheezed and heard my voice reverb on high, like kickback from a mic too close to an amp. It scared me into awareness. Desperately trying to catch my breath, I screamed as I had never before, and in frustration, I sobbed.

I sobbed for what I had heard, what I didn't know, and the confusion I felt.

I sobbed for the woman I was, for the one scared of infertility, and what it meant about me and the rest of my life. In the moment, I knew it, I felt it, I had decided it. "Shannon, you are barren. Therefore, you are broken."

Several years, life coaching, and gut-wrenchingly honest conversations, later, I've learned that the ringing in my ears was tinnitus and can happen in moments of trauma.

I feel labeling infertility as traumatic is accurate. I also feel that symptoms of trauma adequately reflect the last several years of my life; confused, anxious, fearful, depressed, and broken.

Infertility traumatized me. It damaged my relationships, self-esteem and made me a victim. It *changed* me. It also did something unexpected. It taught me the importance of knowing myself. It taught me that at my weakest I wasn't being broken. I was being built.

It allowed me to see that I had no tolerance for struggle. I wanted to be strong and have everything under control, but I was convinced vulnerability as opposite of that. Maybe, right now, you feel the same way, too?

God forbid, we don't have our shit together.

God forbid, we travel a dark road that doesn't end in a 'happily ever after', but grants us the lesson of our lives.

Infertility taught me that I had no bandwidth for strong emotion; that there was no time for sadness, anger, or hurt.

It taught me that I had become conditioned to not feel 'bad'.

It taught me that despite trying to be unaffected by the human condition, I am in fact human, and I get to stop pretending everything is great, when it feels like a stinking pile of crap.

It taught me that I was afraid of vulnerability and believed that logic or science could solve anything. I believed that everything was 'figure-out-able'. However, I didn't take into consideration the impact of figuring out what infertility means to me, and how navigating it, babies, baby-showers, social media posts, and the pain Mother's Day can bring for those who struggle with infertility.

When I first started sharing my experiences about life, life coaching, depression, and infertility on social media, I did it because I couldn't find anyone who was humanizing struggle. There appeared to be no one out there talking about emotion, trauma, and depression, of which I was deep in all three. I wanted to create a dialogue that made it less taboo to discuss our response to it and create a community in which it was safe to share our experiences. Infertility, and my intense response to it, was my taboo topic.

Infertility nearly killed me, my marriage, and every relationship I had. I was trapped inside the intensity of desperately wanting to carry my own child, but plagued by living in the fallout of what it was doing to me, my life, and my body.

I was sick and tired of hearing the same general messages about infertility: "Don't give up", "keep going", "God will bless you when the time is right," while my body was being ravaged to the point of unrecognition, with drastic weight loss, hair loss, cystic acne, pain, and insomnia from the fertility medications.

Everywhere I looked, someone or something was cheering me not to quit. Meanwhile, my consciousness was begging me to consider something different.

I don't blame doctors, family, or friends for their optimism. I understand the intention of cheerleaders. I should. I was one from ages six to eighteen. However, after four years of failed fertility treatments, debt in excess of the thousands, and laparoscopic surgery which revealed a benign tumor, PCOS and stage IV rectovaginal endometriosis, I was tired. I was depressed. I wasn't broken, but I was *really* tired of feeling that way.

I had become someone who was afraid of everything. I had intense anxiety around my period. Sex became a chore, and, my arms and stomach were a breeding ground for bruises.

I hated myself and my body. I hated people with babies. I hated the words uterus and sperm. I was suicidal and I not only *wanted* to quit, I *needed* to, but all the cheerleading brought on a tremendous amount of guilt, so I couldn't.

I felt guilty for wanting to quit fertility treatments. I felt guilty for wanting to feel strong and happy again. I felt guilty for having an opinion. I felt guilty for sharing what was on my heart and in my mind, for fear of hurting or offending someone. I felt guilt, because my intention in a thousand lifetimes is never to hurt or disparage anyone, *ever*, but who am I if I am not living as myself? Who am I if I'm operating from a place that is for other people and not me? Who am I—I am everything but *me*. In fact, if I'm doing everything for the sake of other people, then I'm more *them* than me. Are you more of them than you? Have you ever felt guilty for wanting to say, "No, I've had enough?"

I felt wrong speaking out about our choice to focus on my wellness and cease fertility treatments. Yet, simultaneously, I felt plagued with knowing it as my truth. I wanted to feel empowered to own how we were experiencing infertility and scared of admitting to it at the same time. It's a complex and tangled web, self-awareness. It's like vomiting.

When one feels like they have to vomit, if you're like me, you'll try to talk yourself out of it. "You're not sick." "It's okay, just breathe in through your nose and out through your mouth. It'll go away." "Eat some crackers or Ginger ale? Do we have Ginger ale!?"

Biologically, when you need to vomit, everything in you is telling you to throw-up, yet, we try desperately to hold it in. We don't want to do it. We don't want to do it because it feels uncomfortable and it's usually a sign that we're going to be sick.

Human beings do not want to be uncomfortable or sick. We don't like it. Being uncomfortable is unpredictable and being sick… well, who has time for that?

However, have you ever thrown-up and it felt good? Literally, you vomit and two seconds later you think *Woah, I needed that*! Then, you go about your merry day.

All the potential discomfort and fear of sickness leaves, and low-and-behold, the biological signals we were receiving become okay. They become okay because we're beyond the hairy-scary parts, and on to what we like, know, and feels good, again. Basically, this is the human experience in a nutshell.

We walk around day-after-day, looking at things as comfortable or not, good or bad, and make decisions based on that. When we don't make the decision, is generally because we're thinking and weighing the odds.

The kicker is that life does not respond to us when we say, "Could you hold, please? I need to belabor over feelings or ideas for just a few decades more?" Or, "Excuse me. I didn't order this."

No. Life says, "Hold onto your butts because this shit is going down!" Then, you vomit and wait half a beat before deciding if you're sick or if you've just thrown up to get rid of something nasty. That's how I felt when I started writing and sharing my thoughts and feelings about infertility.

Life kept tugging at me with topics that were giving me a bellyache to share. I had this insatiable urge to be vulnerable, but doing so made me uncomfortable because I was afraid people would think I was telling them not to pursue fertility treatment.

That I was encouraging them to abandon hope. It made me nauseous to do it, but also not do it.

I tried desperately to hold my thoughts in because I was afraid of the backlash or potential to have someone misunderstand me. Instead of being misunderstood by the world, I chose to understand me. I chose it without knowing whether or not I would actually be understood.

I danced in the fuckery of it all for quite some time until I couldn't take it anymore. I pulled the trigger, word vomited all over myself, and everyone else, and discovered that there were more people who understood me, related, and — gasp — *liked* what I had to say. Even better, I felt like me doing it!

I liked the release. I liked the liberty. I liked feeling me come back. I liked the freedom and complexity of sharing, because it required that I become curious, attuned to, and interested in just that. It required that for each thought, feeling, or share I had, that I discover who I was about each of them.

I guess that's how I've learned to do more than just cope with being around babies, baby showers, pregnant woman, and survive Mother's Day. I've learned to distinguish who I wanted to be about each of them.

Do you want to be the kind of woman who glares at babies?

Do you want to be a woman who cries at baby showers?

Do you want to mock pregnancy announcements or posts?

Do you want to fear Mother's Day?

I've forced myself to face being a childless mother. I've forced myself to accept the feelings that come up when I am in social situations where pregnancy or children are discussed. I've challenged myself to notice when I eye-roll people who post about their kids. But, of all this, facing the fact that I chose to accept a future in which I will remain a childless mother has made Mother's Day my biggest challenge.

I love my mom. She is quite possibly the best human on the planet. So, when I noticed that I was celebrating her on Mother's Day in a lackluster way, it jarred me, but also showed me how deeply the holiday was affecting me. I was so deep in my emotional trauma of infertility that not only was I unable to show the genuine depth of my appreciation for her on a deserved, celebratory, day, but I was making it all about me and what I lacked.

The first time I realized this was after we had just agreed to cease fertility treatments. I remember crying most of the day, in between family outings, in the bathroom at the restaurant in which my family was celebrating mom, and that night, as I went to sleep.

The second time I realized Mother's Day as difficult was a year later. I yelled at my husband for not buying me a Mother's Day gift. I justified wanting it by pointing out that I was the mother of our two fur babies. For the record, I still agree with this.

The next time I recall was three years later. My period was late. I was in the all familiar territory of bargaining and praying to God, the Universe, Satan, and Mother Nature, that this Mother's Day I would get my miracle baby. I got my period that very night and consumed an entire bottle of wine in response to it.

The last time I remember being jarred by Mother's Day was right after someone close to me had a baby and again, my period was late. I remember seeing her and everyone around her celebrating her first Mother's Day with such joy, but not me. I was envious and jealous. I wanted to feel the joy, but deep in my heart was the same familiar feeling of focusing on me and how I never would. Again, I got my period that very night. Only this time, I accepted it. I took a long hot bath, let my mind wander to investigate my feelings about it. I sorted through thoughts about who I wanted to be about infertility, babies, Mother's Day and all things related. I became curious about who I was being about all these things and that night, I did not cry myself to sleep.

Sunday, May 12, 2019, was Mother's Day. For the first time in years, I was unbothered. I didn't feel slighted, angry, resentful or left out. I was me.

I called my mom and celebrated her with some flowers. I went to brunch with one mother-in-law and spent the afternoon laughing with another. The entire day was not filled with thoughts of, *Why me, why not us, I am mad, I want to cry*, or feeling like I need to justify, explain, or solve a problem about *me*; how I'm broken, wronged by life, hate that there is an actual day that celebrates the very thing I cannot biologically achieve, or will only ever feel half as happy in my existence, because I will never be a woman who births a child. For the first time in a long time, it wasn't about me and what I lacked.

Let me be the first to tell you, not feeling 'Mother's Day' the way I have felt it in the past was weird. It was *really* fucking weird. But it was also nice.

I woke up the morning after, and the words, "you lived" instead of "you survived" came rushing to me. I felt new and unfamiliar. I felt release and ease. I felt curious about what had changed within me to evoke feeling this way.

I remember crying tears of joy and thinking, *You did it!* I had detangled myself from seeing who I am, as in any way shape or form, defined by this disease. I had stopped making Mother's Day about me in a negative way. That being a mother never did or ever would wholly define me. That I am so much more than this struggle. That I have my happy back, and not even being a childless mother on Mother's Day can disrupt that. It is liberating. It is scary. It takes my breath away. It is nice.

Seeing my new reaction to Mother's Day gave me a great deal of pause and curiosity.

Did I abandon you? The woman who felt controlled and defined by life's hardship.

How can I honor you? The spirit and soul that never gave up and brought me here.

What do I do? I'm scared to forget where I came from and how hard it has been.

Where do I go now? I don't want to be the woman who feels she needs to struggle to become happy with who she was always meant to be. Have you ever asked yourself these questions? Try and see what answers come up.

In my self-inquisition, what I realized is that I got here because I decided I would and so I *am*.

I wanted to become a woman who could see a baby announcement and not cry. I AM.

I wanted to become someone who is happy for others. I AM.

I wanted to become someone who helps others through their human experience. I AM.

I wanted to become someone who could see a baby, attend a baby shower, smile at a pregnant woman, and live through Mother's Day without making it something negative about me. I wanted to see my choice to cease fertility treatments and this holiday as something other than a personal attack. I wanted to see all of it as something other than highlighting my inadequacies, hurts, shame, blame or guilt of the things I was not. I AM.

I wanted to stop being angry at how life turned out for me. I wanted to be happy again. I wanted to have a genuine giggle and stop connecting everything I did or did not do back to infertility.

So, I decided to stop making infertility the epicenter of my existence and make me the most important thing in my life, instead. What position does your well-being hold in your life?

The only way that I could find to courageously do that, know that I am so much more than this disease, was to get vulnerable and intentional in supporting my own self-worth. To make me, and my mental and emotional health, the biggest priority in my life. It was to put me first, see how mean and disparaging I was being to myself, see how my every move in life was influenced by infertility, and believe that this *thing* does not get to control me. I say what goes, and what I decided to get me here is that I am willing to believe that we get to be built by our struggle.

Now, I know that I am a woman who lived through what nearly destroyed her to discover it created her. I know that I am someone who faced what felt bigger than her to decide that I am responsible for my thoughts. I also know that I don't want to be that woman *ever* again if I don't have to be. Let me be clear, *we* don't have to be. Are you willing to believe that for yourself?

I want to be a woman who does not have to experience a massive struggle to find who she is. What are you curious to learn about you?

I want to be a woman who decides that self-discovery gets to feel light, airy, sparkly, and magical. Where is there room for ease in your life?

I want to be a woman who knows what her body cannot do without contempt, so as to celebrate and love it for all that it can. What relationship are you in with your body?

I want to be a woman who can enjoy the pleasure and desire for sex, instead of seeing it as a means to an end. What is sex and pleasure like for you?

I want to be a woman who knows that when I am loving myself with a truthful, responsible, and intentional love, that I not only respond to me with compassion and understanding, but that it enables me to do the same for everyone I encounter. What intentions do you hold for yourself?

I, also, want to be a woman who knows that struggle is human and humanizing it is about the most healing thing we can do for ourselves. How are you humanizing who you are in your struggles?

I know that it is this thinking, plus, my choice to be a childless Mother, that brings me guilt. I also know that feeling guilty is a choice.

Wanting and believing a journey can be easy are not the same thing. How do I know? Look at the way I've described my sharing process. In case you forgot, I compared it to vomiting. Vomiting! Literally, the thing I like the least in the world. The *least*. Over spiders, coconut, and metal being shoved into my vagina. Vomiting reigns supreme!

So, yes. Waking up one-day, after years of struggling with infertility, to discover a day that had consistently tormented me no longer had that effect was quite confusing. But, I, and you, are both smart enough to know that it didn't just happen in one day. It happened over many days, experiences, and with an intentional knowing that being someone who was leveled by pregnancy, children, and motherhood is not someone I wanted to be. Is that the intention of who you want to be?

Yes. To me, it makes sense that I would face this new and non-reactionary response with guilt instead of jubilation, celebration, gratitude, and release. It makes sense, because I've lived with guilt about not being able to get pregnant for so long, that to suddenly have it all change, made me feel guilty about not feeling guilty. It made me feel self-righteous for no longer beating myself up over what my body cannot do. Are you ridden with feelings of guilt about wanting to heal your relationship to self?

Yes. To me, it is overwhelming to admit and share my guilt about revealing that I have worked to heal myself. Because, for so long, I chose to see the discomfort as natural and justified. I chose to feel right in anger about what women are biologically sold our bodies are *supposed* to do. I chose to feel alienated from myself and society because I couldn't get what I wanted and saw as my human right. What are you looking to be right about?

I feel guilty because for four years, I let infertility consume me and who I was in my life. But, the truth is, it is what happened. Infertility became bigger than me. It became more important than me. It made all the decisions. It decided if I was happy, sad, angry, or jubilant. It decided if I was worthy or not. It ruled me and it ruled who I was to the world. Are you letting infertility mean more to you than you?

Infertility is the struggle of my life. If it is the struggle of yours, please know that I see you, I hear you, and I feel you on a soul level that makes me want to stand up and scream before a crowd of other infertility warriors, like us, "YOU ARE MORE THAN THIS." And, ask, "What is this moment teaching you?"

It has taught me countless lessons about relationships, responsibility, emotional intelligence, creativity, and humans. It has taught me about compassion and boundaries. It has taught me that while I did not get to bear or birth my biological child, that does not define me, and it only does if I let it. Are you letting infertility and your ability, or lack thereof, define you?

I believe infertility will continue to teach me until my end of days, and while continuing to discern its teachings, I don't pretend that there can't or won't be other struggles in life. However, in the process of seeing the lessons of our lives, I know that I'd rather not have my history repeat itself. That my intention is to see every struggle, trial or tribulation, as something from which I am meant to learn. That in order to learn how to love and experience all the amazing attributes of myself on this planet, I have to be a good student to my story. I have to let myself feel and think as I need to, but with the understanding that I am the star of my life and my goal is to operate from a place that supports it.

After all this time, struggle, depression, and self-destructive thinking, feeling, and action, I have breached the castle walls. I have penetrated the fortress I built around myself that locked me in and made me believe that in Shannon's life, her way will always be the hard way. I have changed the narrative for me to see that I am tired of the same old story. I already know how it ends. 50% of the time shit goes my way and 50% of the time it doesn't. So, why not focus on what I want more than putting an energy out into the universe that is always trying to discern how to react when it doesn't go my way?

What if we allowed for the human in a struggle to be the most important part?

What if we stopped seeing ourselves as broken?

What then?

I'll tell you what, shit starts to feel like magic every fucking day.

Life starts to feel like no matter what happens you can handle it.

Failure starts to seem like not that big of a deal.

And, fear, well, fuck that bitch, she's got nothing on determination and courage.

You start to become your most trusted ally and resource on this planet when you allow You to be you with ease.

You start to see that you didn't do anything wrong. With infertility, you don't deserve the pain you're in and therefore, you do not have to beat yourself up over it.

You start to see that you are bigger than your struggle.

On Mother's Day, I found myself—a new self. How ironic, to discover rebirth, through self-awareness with ease on a day that used to make me feel defeated. How incredible, to experience a day that used to terrorize me with new thoughts and feelings. How freeing, to see that in the middle of living your everyday, deciding who you want to be requires that you be it. Have you decided who you want to be about your life?

I don't know what the future holds for me, but I know that the experiences of my life will lead me to it, because I know who I want to be about my life. I also know that when the future becomes the present, I will not be meeting the second, third or fourth version of myself. I don't know how many iterations there will be, but I know that regardless of the levity or severity of life's circumstances, with ease, I am already excited to meet her and what she has to teach me, because I, and you, are never being broken. If we are willing to see that every journey comes with a lesson designed to teach us about ourselves, then the more we intentionally pursue this thinking, we are able to see into the heart of who we want to be about our experiences. We are able to see that we are never broken, we are only ever being built.

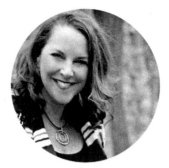

Dana Zarcone, MSCC, NBCC, CEP

Dana Zarcone, the founder of Dana Zarcone International, LLC., runs a successful coaching, consulting and publishing company that focuses on helping clients break through barriers, unleash their full potential and become an unstoppable force in life and business!

Leveraging her twenty-five-year corporate career and certifications as a master trainer, national board-certified counselor, and energy psychologist, Dana provides local and virtual services that include experiential workshops, training classes and individual and group coaching. In addition, Dana is a 6X #1 international bestselling author, a highly sought-after publisher, motivational speaker, and podcast host.

Dana integrates neuroscience, quantum physics, kinesiology, and psychology to show her clients what is truly possible. Through her broad range of education, research, and experience, she has developed a revolutionary approach that has helped hundreds of clients around the world break through barriers and become the badass they were born to be!

Want to publish your story? Connect with her today!

Connect with Dana:
www.DanaZarcone.com
https://www.facebook.com/danazarcone
https://www.facebook.com/groups/healyourselfhappy/
https://www.instagram.com/dana_zarcone/

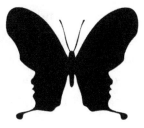

The Willingness to Surrender

By Dana Zarcone

My husband and I got married later in life. We were forty and thirty-three, respectively. You'd think that we'd have jumped on the baby bandwagon as soon as possible. Not so for us. We were both in the prime of our careers, entertaining customers, traveling all over the world, going on weekend excursions in our boat.

In addition to my corporate career, I had my private practice as a national board-certified counselor and I was a group fitness instructor for the local YMCA. Needless to say, we were enjoying life to the fullest. We talked about having kids 'one day' but we weren't in any hurry. Truth be told, we weren't even sure we really wanted kids.

I had girl friends that were older than I was that were trying to have kids. They felt the maternal instinct that I was lacking at the time. Once they started trying, some were fortunate enough to get pregnant right away. Some, unfortunately, were not. One friend found out that she had severe endometriosis and getting pregnant would be almost impossible. She and her husband decided to adopt.

Another discovered that she wouldn't be able to get pregnant without the help of in-vitro fertilization. She so desperately wanted to have kids of her own but didn't want to adopt because she wanted to be pregnant. So she and her husband decided to go for it. Each IVF treatment cost around $10,000. They did it at least four times. Over the course of a couple of years, I watched her go on this emotional roller coaster, bracing for the bad news once again until, finally, she ended up pregnant and gave birth to a beautiful boy.

It always puzzled me how someone could want so desperately to be pregnant. *I mean really?* Who in their right mind would be so desperate to be pregnant that they'd choose to experience severe morning sickness, painful swelling of your breasts, nausea, fatigue and all the other symptoms that go with it?!

For me, this was odd. How can someone want to be pregnant so badly? How can someone want to be a mother so badly? I was a bit baffled. As I mentioned, I didn't feel the maternal instinct like most of my friends. I watched them go through years of promises, heartbreak, failures, and successes… I didn't want it that bad. I just didn't.

As I mentioned, my husband and I got married later in life. We were really enjoying our freedom. Especially being a couple that could travel the world on our company's dime, embark on amazing adventures and come home to our quiet sanctuary. That said, we realized that we were taking the idea of potential parenthood for granted. We were assuming that if we decided to have kids one day that it'd be easy. But, what if it wasn't? What if we had to struggle like so many of our friends?

These questions begged some real soul searching for both of us. *Do we really want kids?* Honestly, we weren't entirely sure. So we decided that we would put the decision in God's hands. We wouldn't try, per se, but if it happened then it must be what is meant to be. So, I went off the pill.

About six weeks later, I had some of those terrible symptoms. My breasts were tender, I was nauseous and certain smells made me want to vomit. And, yes, I was two weeks late—I'm *never* late! So many thoughts began to race through my mind. *Are you kidding me?! Could this really be happening? Oh shit! I'm not sure I'm ready for this!* But, I needed to know so off to the drug store I went!

That night, I took my first pregnancy test ever. As my husband and I waited for the results, the tension started to build. Each passing minute felt like an hour. My mind was racing with all the possible ways my life would never be the same. This would be a defining moment. I took a long, deep breath, picked up the test strip and there it was. Two dark lines indicating that I was, indeed, pregnant.

My husband threw both of his hands in the air and shouted, "Woo-hoo! We're having a baby!" Me on the other hand... I sat there stunned, panic-stricken, gasping for air as I tried to choke back the tears. Only these weren't happy tears. I wasn't happy at all! I felt as if I had just been sentenced to life in prison! Our weekend excursions, carefree travel, boating... over! My private practice... over! Our lives would only be about sleepless nights, poopy, smelly diapers, and temper tantrums! Our lives would never be the same again!

It took me a couple of weeks to come to grips that we made the decision to 'let go and let God', and God had spoken loud and clear! There was a part of me that was feeling horribly guilty. Especially after watching so many of our friends try so desperately to have kids only to end up heartbroken. Here I was, unsure if I really wanted a child after getting pregnant so easily and effortlessly.

I was fortunate in that the pregnancy was a breeze. No morning sickness. No nausea to speak of. In fact, I was just 'getting bigger'! I was often told that I had that new mother glow! I was full of energy... more energy than I would usually have. *Wow! Pregnancy isn't so bad after all!* I said to myself.

I began to read every book I could about pregnancy and becoming a mother. Frankly, I was in awe realizing that my husband and I were able to create another human being. *How is this even possible? It is truly a miracle that we can procreate.* Frankly, I'm still in awe of this fact! I understand the science behind it but when you really think about it... isn't it crazy that we can create another human being?!

Wow and holy cow! I have a little human being growing inside of me! I began to embrace the idea of being a mother and, dare I say, I was becoming excited. I was learning everything I could about the development of my baby and what my life was going to be like as a new mother.

As every first-time parents would do, we started shopping for furniture, looking at all the different styles of cribs, changing tables and rocking chairs. We were avid boaters, so it was a no brainer that our nursery would have a nautical theme. We bought wallpaper boarder, crib bumpers, lamps, and a musical mobile... everything we needed to create a warm, welcoming environment for our new baby.

Oh... my ... God! I'm going to be a mother! I can't wait!

Family and friends were just as excited as we were. My mother, in particular, as she was pushing us to have a baby for years! She was frustrated we waited so long and couldn't wait to be a grandmother! At the time, I was thirty-eight years old.

As a result of my age, I had to go to a geneticist to assess potential risks. During my appointment, my doctor had to leave the room. Out of curiosity, I leaned over the desk to take a peek at my file and there it was highlighted in yellow highlighter... 'Elderly mother'! *Elderly mother?!* What the heck! I was only thirty-eight for goodness sakes! Now, they use the politically correct term of 'advanced maternal age'. Either way, I was being classified as an old mother. That, in and of itself, was an eye-opener.

Being an older mother meant there was a greater potential for complications for both me and the baby. But, at the time, I was in the best shape of my life. The year before, my husband and I ran the Marine Corps marathon in Washington, D.C., I was teaching four to five fitness classes a week and I worked out every day that I wasn't teaching a class. My pregnancy was effortless and I was fit and fab at the time! So, what could possibly go wrong?

Mother's Day was quickly approaching. My first Mother's Day as a mother. I couldn't wait! My husband was always a romantic guy so he had all kinds of fun things planned. In fact, I'm not sure who was more excited… me or him? On that day, I was sixteen weeks along, almost halfway to the finish line. My belly was getting big and I was starting to experience some movement, making motherhood seem more real than ever.

It was mid-afternoon when I went to the bathroom and everything changed. As I stood up to flush I looked down and saw a lot of blood! My knees grew weak, my chest tightened, my throat tried to close up as I started to scream. My body riddled with chills, the whole house started to spin as a flood of tears consumed my eyes, blurring my vision.

Then and there, I knew. I could feel it… the emptiness in my heart, the lifeless feeling in my belly. *I'm not pregnant anymore. I knew at that moment; I lost my baby. I was devastated. How is this happening to me? What went wrong? How am I going to tell my husband? Oh my God. How am I going to tell my husband?!*

I think he could sense something was wrong. Why was I taking so long? So he came upstairs to check on me. He took one look at me and started to cry. Just as I did, he knew what had happened. Our baby was taken from us. We weren't going to be parents after all.

Being so far along, we had fallen in love with the baby and the idea of being parents. I think we even fell in love with the idea of getting very little sleep and changing poopy, smelly diapers! Now the thought of a good night's sleep without the two o'clock feedings made me extremely sad.

The next day, I called my OBGYN and she had me come in that day. She confirmed that I wasn't carrying a viable fetus anymore. I felt like such a failure. We never should have waited so long. Now, because I was an 'elderly mother' I was unable to carry a baby to term and give my husband a child.

I found it ironic that when I first became pregnant, I cried because being pregnant meant that I was condemned to a life sentence of responsibilities that I wasn't prepared to assume. Then, the day I miscarried, I cried because I was in love and wanted nothing more than to hold that baby in my arms. I wanted nothing more than to be a mother.

Needless to say, I was in mourning. I was grieving. Both of us were grieving in our own ways. I cried a lot and, frankly, felt so alone. Most of my friends had children by then. I couldn't bear to be around them because it was too painful. And, I couldn't tell them because I was too ashamed. Eventually, they'd find out though, because it was no secret that we were expecting.

At the time, I had just graduated from the Institute of Core Energetics, where I had become certified as an energy psychologist. I decided to tell my classmates what had happened. The institute is located in New York City but all of us who attended live all over the place. So, I really didn't have anyone locally I could look to for support. One of my classmates came up with the idea of having a 'virtual service' where we would all come together to pray for a half-hour on a specific date and time.

My husband and I went into the nursery, lit a candle, closed our eyes, and centered ourselves. As time elapsed, I was feeling more and more consumed with love, light, and energy. It was unlike anything I had ever experienced before. I felt so loved and supported. My heart opened and I began to sob. I sobbed because I was in tune with how much gratitude I felt towards my classmates who took the time to 'be with me' that afternoon. I sobbed because I was going to miss this baby so much. But what's more amazing is that I sobbed because I was filled with gratitude for this baby coming into my life.

As we sat there in silence, in prayer, I knew in my heart that I was pregnant with a baby boy. He was a tremendous blessing in my life. In just sixteen weeks, he taught me about what it meant to be a mother and that I really did want to be one. He taught me that it meant to be responsible for another human being. That I was more capable of loving someone else than I had ever thought possible. This baby was a huge blessing and I know with all my heart that this is why he came into my life. To teach me that I was meant for motherhood.

Just over a year later, I was blessed with a beautiful baby girl. We are now the proud parents of two amazing young ladies, a fifteen and eleven-year-old. They know that they have a baby brother who is in heaven watching over them. They know that it's because of him that I am able to love my daughters with all my heart... more than I ever thought possible.

This experience taught me a lot about life. It taught me that amazing things can come into your life if you're willing to surrender to what God and the universe have in store for you. It taught me that, even some of the most tragic experiences are meant to teach us something about ourselves – our resistance to life, our limitations and, more importantly, our full potential!

I'm in awe right now because as I am finishing this chapter, I look over at the clock to see what time it is. It is 11:11 a.m. Seems like every time I look at the clock it's 11:11. This is my sign that those who've passed before me —including my son— are connected to me, protecting me and sending me a ton of love and light. It reminds me that we are all connected. We are all one. We are all love.

Until we meet again, my angels.

Conclusion

Your journey with Silent Grief, Healing, and Hope has come to an end.

I am very proud of the authors that contributed to this book! Their vulnerability has not gone unnoticed. These authors not only wrote about their struggles with infertility, having a miscarriage or losing a child, but relived and struggled heartache and pain to bring this book to life.

It is my hope that you were able to relate to the writers and found a piece of yourself in these stories as the writer experienced their own challenging times of grief and loss. If you are currently suffering in a similar manner, I hope this book brings you peace, comfort, and support.

Grief has no beginning or end. Losing a child, experiencing a miscarriage or struggling to become pregnant are true misgivings. Regardless of our beliefs or experiences, we all need to learn and revisit self-love and process our emotions. This book is one support network that you may need.

Being a counselor, I know far too well the benefits of self-talk and processing our emotions fully.

If you are in counseling or attend a support group, I praise you for taking that leap to reach out for your personal needs and growth. If you are questioning extra support for any part of your life, please make the phone call or walk into a counseling office to see how a professional may be able to help you.

I want to thank you, the reader, for choosing this book. We would all love for you to go to our Amazon listing and write a personal review. This would give our writers additional support, and provide valuable information for future readers! Thank you again for all of your support!

Remember to make today lovely, express gratitude and carry hope.

Sincerely,

Danielle Lynn

Addictions counselor, bestselling author, health & wellness coach, Christian life coach.

www.daniellelynninspires.com

CPSIA information can be obtained
at www.ICGtesting.com
Printed in the USA
BVHW042100010421
603964BV00004B/12